the
12-Week
fitness
project

the
12-Week
fitness
project

RUJUTA
DIWEKAR

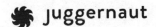 juggernaut

JUGGERNAUT BOOKS

KS House, 118 Shahpur Jat, New Delhi 110049, India

First published by Juggernaut Books 2020

10 9 8 7 6 5 4 3 2 1

P-ISBN: 9789353450885
E-ISBN: 9789353450892

Typeset in Adobe Garamond by Haitenlo Semy

Printed and bound in India by Thomson Press India Ltd

Contents

For each guideline

- The guideline
- Notes on how to follow
  (as applicable)
- Benefits or Why to follow
- FAQs

Preface

Health beyond weight loss

Like all good things the #12weekfitnessproject was born spontaneously.

And like all things spontaneous, this one too had a long history. In fact, you could say that this project arose because, as a nutritionist and fitness professional, I have seen history repeat itself time and time again. Of people resolving to get fit every year, committing to eating right, exercising, and then all of it fizzling out in about six weeks. Life, as they say, takes over.

But that is only if you think of health and fitness as separate from living your life. The fitness project was born out of the idea that health and fitness were and should be thought of as an integral part of life. A fitness plan that was so effortless, so common sense, so organic that you could make permanent, lasting changes to your life without turning it upside down. An evolution of yourself. Not an instant revolution.

This idea also chimes with the latest research in nutrition science and was very much in evidence at the prestigious European Nutrition Conference (FENS), held in Dublin in October 2019. The FENS is like the Olympics of nutrition conferences and happens every four years. It's a place of learning, sharing and exploring the latest that this interesting field of food and nutrition has to offer. We presented the findings of the 12-week fitness project at the conference, marking our debut on the international scene with a very desi approach to food, health and lifestyle.

So, to keep it short, here's what the latest in nutrition science has to say:

- About 25%–30% of obese population is healthy, that is, they are MHO – metabolically healthy obese.
- This means that they have no or very low risk to diabetes, cancer, heart disease, etc., and have their liver fat and lipid profile under control.
- But the narrative around health is heavily misinformed and entirely tilted in favour of the weighing scales.
- Because of this the most common advice that you are likely to receive is to lose some weight.

- People then resort to diets that help them quickly lose that weight.
- Most, if not all, diets that people adopt use restrictions on either calories, food groups, timings or portions.
- This means that most people have embarked on an unsustainable weight loss journey.
- They invariably fall off this regime, resume their normal lifestyle and the weight creeps back with a vengeance.
- And now here's the scary part. The moment this happens, they are 150% more likely to get a lifestyle disease like diabetes, cancer, heart disease, etc., than when they were earlier at the same weight.
- Essentially, a more sustainable approach to health is recommended instead of a more drastic approach.
- As far as health risks go, body weight loss of 5%–10% over a year is considered sustainable.
- The key is to form diet and workout habits that lead to long-lasting changes to lifestyle and to long-term improvements in health and well-being.

- A sustainable diet should be comprised of food that meets these three essential criteria – it should be rich in nutrients, culturally resonant and ecologically sensitive.
- Simply put, eat local, seasonal and traditional, and invest in health with a long-term approach.

In a way, it seems that science is making a full U-turn to be on the same page as that of your grandmom's food wisdom. But truth be told, nutrition science has been steadily, although slowly, been refining its approach to health and well-being. But now you can officially say that food as a sum total of carbs, protein and fat is a thing of the past.

Nutrition science has realized that, in its full potential, food doesn't just make people healthy but it can lead to a resurgence in the local economy and revive or at least help global ecology recover. Not a bad mix of tradition, common sense and science, I would say.

But then this is the stuff that we all already know. We have observed and suffered the short-term fixes and the long-term health consequences in our own bodies and of those around us. We have also seen way too often how one thing is blamed for all the troubles that we face with our weight.

If fat was the bad boy 20 years ago, carbs are the new monster, but the promise is the same old one. Remove this one ingredient from your life and you will be healthy. The fitness project was born out of the need to cut through this narrative and to build a more sustainable, sensible and scientific approach to health.

It's like we all want to be swept off our feet by the man who will come into our life in his fancy sports car and James Bond smile but we all know that the one for keeps is the one who reminds you to pack your toothbrush in your travel kit when you have forgotten to do so. This fitness project is going to be that guy for you. Your steady, strong, silent companion, your guide to sustainable fitness.

Here's to brand-new you.

Chapter 1

About the 12-week fitness project

The 12-week fitness project is special for many reasons. One of the reasons is the response it received. Within 5 minutes of opening up registration, 500 people had signed up.

'Should I close it?' I asked my partner, GP, while sitting on my balcony, sipping chai. 'No, dekhte hain,' he replied. 'Let's wait for 5000.' I thought we would hit that number by the next morning. It was about 5 or 5.30 p.m. In the next hour, we had hit 5000 and by the next morning we had 75,000. We were overwhelmed, to say the least. We closed the forms and my office phone started ringing off the hook.

'Rujuta Diwekar's office,' I said, answering one of the calls. 'What's wrong with her?' asked the voice on the line. 'Why are the forms closed?' 'Sir, we have about 75,000 registrations.' 'So? You will close it? Is it some sort of punishment for people who are not constantly glued to FB on their phones?' 'No,' I managed. 'We won't be able to deal with so many people or track their parameters.'

'See,' he retorted, 'that's the problem with people like Rujuta. Scalability se darte hain. They underuse technology. There are people right here in my office in Hyderabad, ten guys at least on my floor, who can crunch that data for you. What do you plan to do with the data?' 'Just use it to track progress,' I answered.

'Then use technology, madam, open those forms. Let this advice get to people, rarely do these kinds of things come by for free. Don't let your lack of vision ruin it. Take 25,000 to 35,000 more registrations and then tell people that they can still follow the guidelines but not officially be part of the project. Ek critical mass toh pahunchne do.' Shit! Thank you for that earful, I wanted to say, but I hung up and did exactly as directed.

At the end of 12 weeks, with 1.25 lakh+ participants from 40+ countries filling out compliance forms every week and marking their progress on health parameters every month, everyone I knew in IT wanted to know how I was going to analyse the data that was pouring in.

'Do you have people who can do it? What program are you using?' We had no clue. We knew from the summary given by Google forms that there had been huge improvement in health parameters and inch loss from waist, but we didn't know how to get the exact numbers.

Thankfully for us, Vikas Singh from MyGov and Dhawal Goyal, an engineer from IIT Bombay, came to our rescue and volunteered to help us with the analysis. This data crunching was a big part of the fitness project and without them the impact of the fitness project would never have been quantitatively measured.

We would know it had worked – we knew that in our hearts – but exactly how much and how well we would never have known. So, Vikas and Dhawal, this is not the acknowledgements page, but you are my angels, thank you. It's a rare opportunity to track free, living individuals in a real-life setting and this wouldn't have been possible without you.

Also, to all our participants, thank you for following the guidelines, tracking your parameters and sharing your progress every week. Especially the 1500 who didn't miss filling and sharing even a single form. You guys are the gods of this project. To each one of you who participated, thank you, and know that the biggest universities and the most acclaimed of researchers have to pay people to be part of such projects. You did this for free, your love and your support is *the* most special aspect of the project. I will carry your debt in my heart forever.

Note: The project report has now been published as a research paper in an international public health journal and you can access and cite it as follows:
'Culturally relevant food and lifestyle interventions lead to sustainable public health'. *Proceedings of the International Conference on Public Health*, 5(1): 21–26.
https://doi.org/10.17501/23246735.2019.5103

Who, why and how of the project

We live in times of food confusion. For simple questions like 'how can I stay healthy?', 'what should I eat?' there are tons of complicated answers, most of them contradicting each other. This is also evident in the rise of diet trends globally, even as public health continues to deteriorate.

In India, we now have a huge population that suffers from non-communicable diseases (NCDs), like obesity, diabetes, cancer, PCOD, heart ailments, mental health issues, etc. Where does nutrition science stand on this? Well, the latest in nutrition science says that culturally relevant foods and eating practices are the gold standard for good nutrition. In other words, **the time-tested wisdom of your grandmother, passed down over generations, is what you should go by.**

So what does culturally relevant foods and eating practices mean in our day-to-day lives? Simply, it means we should eat local, seasonal and traditional. Eating local means eating rice and not quinoa. Eating seasonal means eating guava in winter and mango in summer, and not kiwi throughout the year. **Eating traditional means following the wisdom of our grandmothers in totality. So haldi in tadka and not as a supplement. We have to bring back the pride in our culture, our languages and our cuisine.**

So that's why this project – because fitness is uncomplicated, inexpensive and something that everyone should have access to.

As to the how

(a) One guideline was given every week, to be followed cumulatively. This meant that in week 2, they followed week 1 guideline + week 2 guideline, and in week 3 = week 1 + 2 + 3, and so on.

(b) At the end of each week, participants noted down their compliance with the guidelines on the following scale – mostly, 50–50, not really.

(c) At the end of each month, they rated their progress on a scale of 1–5 (where higher rating meant better results) on the following metabolic health parameters – energy levels, sleep quality, acidity/indigestion, sweet cravings, exercise compliance and PMS/period pain (for women). They also tracked inch loss at waist.

Who?

Anyone, anywhere, who was willing to make the effort daily for himself/herself. The guidelines had specifications, wherever needed, for lifestyle conditions like diabetes, PCOD, thyroid, etc., and also for which country they lived in.

Results

Here are the improvements the participants recorded.

1. Percentage improvement in metabolic health parameters (based on self-rating by participants on a scale of 1–5)

Metabolic health parameters	Improvement in all participants	Improvement in consistent participants
Energy levels through the day	33%	44%
Sleep quality during the night	31%	41%
Acidity/bloating/indigestion	52%	68%
Sweet cravings after meals	51%	66%
Exercise compliance through the week	44%	54%
Pain during PMS/period (for women)	48%	53%

2. Improvement in individual metabolic health parameters over 12 weeks (self-reported by consistent participants on a scale of 1–5). The numbers in the charts are averages of the ratings.

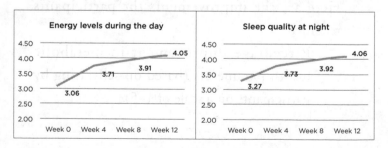

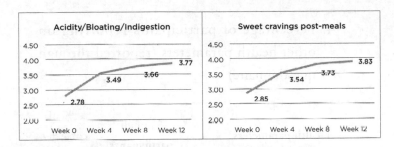

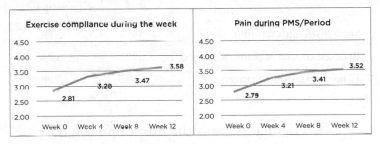

3. Inch loss at the navel

Inch loss at navel	All participants	Consistent participants
Up to 1 inch	38.4%	41.7%
1–2 inches	22.8%	27.8%
>2 inches	12.4%	13.0%
Total	73.6%	82.5%

4. Percentage of participants reporting on other health parameters (reported through questionnaire)

Health parameters	% of all participants	% of consistent participants
Started strength training	56%	62%
Reduced contact of plastic with food	69%	69%
Fitness perception changed	74%	79%

5. Highlights from the questionnaire posed at the end of the year (for sustainability of guidelines)

Questions	% of participants reporting 'yes'
Consistently followed guidelines?	91%
Metabolic health continues to improve?	75%
Developed a positive mindset towards health?	74%
Lost further inches from navel?	70%
No more food fads?	65%

The 12 Week
FITNESS
PROJECT
IMPACT REPORT

Jan-Mar 2018

40+ COUNTRIES
1.25 LAKH PARTICIPANTS
12 WEEKLY GUIDELINES
15000 AVG. WEEKLY FORMS FILLED

Un-complicating Fitness
- Focus on metabolic health parameters, not weight loss.
- Simple to follow, culturally compliant interventions are sustainable.
- Local, seasonal, traditional food; not carbs, proteins, fats and calories.

1. Improvement in metabolic health parameters over 12 weeks

Energy Levels
44% Improvement

Sleep Quality
41% Improvement

Acidity/ Indigestion
68% Improvement

Sweet Cravings
66% Improvement

Exercise Compliance
54% Improvement

PMS/ Period Pain
53% Improvement

2. Better health and habits overall (% of participants)

Inch Loss from waist
83%

Food Perception Improved
80%

Started Strength Training
62%

Reduction in Plastic Use
70%

3. Follow up after 1 year - highlights

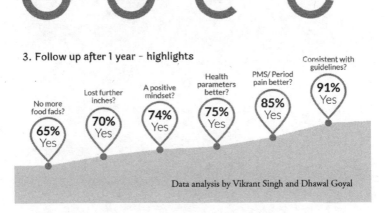

No more food fads?
65% Yes

Lost further inches?
70% Yes

A positive mindset?
74% Yes

Health parameters better?
75% Yes

PMS/ Period pain better?
85% Yes

Consistent with guidelines?
91% Yes

Data analysis by Vikrant Singh and Dhawal Goyal

11

Chapter 2

The three rules of sustainable health

In this chapter, we look at the current diet trends, where they originate from, why they haven't been able to find long-term solutions for our health and well-being, and what you, as an individual, can do for good health and a disease-free life. Specifically, we cover these three rules of sustainable health:

1. Metabolic health vs weight loss
2. All-round vs one-dimensional approach
3. Long-term vs short-term solutions

These rules form the basis of the guidelines that follow in the next section of the book.

Diet trends 2.0

Diet trends don't come and go, they go and come back. As the 2.0 versions of their earlier selves. It's the same old wine, but in a new bottle, amplified via social media, influencers and even apps. So, Atkins or paleo is now keto or LCHF (low carb, high fat) diet. (One of my clients famously called it low on confidence and high on farts to describe how she felt while she was on it.) Low-calorie trends like 5:2 diet from earlier this decade are now intermittent fasting or time-restricted eating, etc. While one urges you to eat like a hunter, the other wants you to fast like your ancestors. Of course, you don't need to hunt while living in a cave and fasting delicacies like sabudana khichdi, sweet potato, samo kheer, singhare ki roti, arbi ki sabzi etc., are not even in the picture. But the noise around the diets drowns these minor details.

It's not that the weight loss and food industry lacks imagination when it comes to introducing revolutionary diet trends. It's just that they are limited by the parameters on the basis of which new diet trends can be developed. Most, if not all, diet trends in the modern era work by either restricting calories (through fewer meals or timings or portions) or reducing/eliminating food groups (counting macros, removing carbs, etc.)

Here is a quick summary.

Types of diet trends	Basic idea	Examples	Cultural spin	Basic flaw
Reduce food groups	Reduce food to carb/protein/fat and then remove or reduce any one of these food groups from the diet while overemphasizing the others	*1.0 trends:* Atkins, South Beach *2.0 trends:* keto, paleo, LCHF	Hunter-gatherer lifestyle	Looks at food from a reductionist view of food groups. Misses the bigger picture which links food to culture, cuisine and crop cycle – the food system approach.
Restrict calories	Restrict intake of calories either by portion control or by eating fewer times or in a limited time window	*1.0 trends:* Low-cal diets, 5:2, 2 meals a day, weight watchers *2.0 trends:* Intermittent fasting, time-restricted eating, juice diet	Ritual fasting, spiritual detox	Calorie counting is unscientific and unsustainable. Fasting as a trend misses the point of ritual fasting which was to add diversity to diets. Eating as per appetite is a time-tested method to stay healthy

So, as an individual who is looking to lead a healthy life, a life free from diseases and disabilities, what can we learn from the story of diet trends? That they are unsustainable. They don't lead to long-term good health, and in fact can cause more harm than good. And that good health doesn't come from following the food industry and influencers, but lies at the heart of our homes – our kitchens. And the people you must listen to are our grandmothers at home and the farmers outside. They are deeply integrated with the food systems, are the bearers of time-tested wisdom and, in the case of your elders, are genuinely invested in your well-being.

Vote for good health

It's very important to understand that health is not just a matter of individual responsibility but our governments and policymakers play a big role too. Take the example of pollution. Science has now conclusively proven that pollution is an independent risk factor for NCDs like diabetes, cancer, heart ailments, etc. This means that even if at an individual level you make all the efforts to eat right, don't smoke or drink alcohol, work out regularly and sleep on time, you are still highly susceptible to developing these diseases just because you live in a polluted city. Another example is policies on advertisement of junk food, especially those targeted at kids, and its impact on their health. Similarly, governments and policymakers can make a big impact on our health by regulating plastic packaging, imposing taxes on junk food, facilitating rural–urban linkages for fresh food, promoting walkable cities with footpaths and green spaces, etc. So what can *you* do? Vote for and demand such policies from your representatives in the government.

There is still a lot you can do at an individual level to ensure sustainable health for yourself and for your family, and that's where this book comes in. But how does one go about deciding if a diet pattern, a workout regime or a lifestyle will lead to good health? Fortunately for us, the latest in nutrition science is on the same page with our traditional food wisdom and common sense on this front. And drawing on this coming together of traditional wisdom with science, I have made three easy rules which can help you decide if you are on the sustainable path to health and fitness.

The three rules of sustainable health

1. **Metabolic health parameters vs weight loss**

   The thing is that even when diet trends come back with a new name and a new game, the basic premise stays the same – weight loss. Sometimes outright, sometimes garnished with words and concepts like detoxify, rejuvenation, anti-diabetes, anti-cancer, etc. But for any diet trend to thrive, weight loss is the central pillar. Ever heard of a viral diet trend whose only promise is 'food security for all' or even a modest one like 'better digestion and no acidity'? The multi-billion-dollar food industry needs our focus to stay on losing weight for it to stay profitable.

   But what we notice in our daily lives, if we pay attention, is that the things that really matter when it comes to our well-being are usually the ones we can't measure on a weighing scale or on a scale of any kind. Do we sleep well at night, do we wake up feeling fresh, do our energy levels stay good through the day, do we suffer from acidity, bloating and indigestion, do we get sweet cravings after meals, are we able to stay active and comply with exercise plans and do we have painful PMS and periods, etc.?

In scientific terminology, the above parameters are surrogate measures of metabolic health. They give an indication of how well your hormones are behaving, how your heart health is, how diverse your gut bacteria are, whether your blood sugar is well regulated, and so much more. In other words, they are markers of your susceptibility to NCDs like diabetes, cancer, PCOD, thyroid conditions, heart ailments, mental health issues, etc. And remember, NCDs account for almost 75% of early deaths worldwide.

And one of the biggest reasons for deteriorating public health, even as diet trends proliferate, is the single-minded focus on losing weight at the cost of metabolic health. The narrative of what accounts for good health therefore has to shift from weight loss to metabolic health.

What your weighing machine doesn't tell you

Body weight is not an indicator of fatness or fitness. It is simply an indicator of yeh bakra kitne mein katega. Madam, we have a New Year package offer going on. You just pay for 5 kg, hum aap ko 2 kg ka loss uss pe free denge. This is all the purpose that the weighing machine serves. Which is why I have never used weighing scales in my work from day one. Some of my clients loved the idea. 'Relaxed lagtey idhar aake,' said one client. At all the places that she had been to earlier for diets, she would first get scolded for not losing enough and then be punished with a stricter diet, much less food and much more of exercise (walking mostly) until the next appointment.

Most diets get you to lose body weight by compromising on your water or muscle and bone density. Which is exactly why you get weaker, sicker and much more irritable with weight loss. Those around you begin to feel that you look sick, and you begin to feel that they are just jealous bitches because you lost 7 kilos over two months.

People lose weight, ya, in war, in sickness, in stress. The key, as Kareena Kapoor says, is to lose weight with a smile and without compromising on your favourite foods. Without losing sleep over it, without losing din ka chain, without losing life ka maza. The idea is to be light on your feet, not on the scales.

And if you are still asking me why everyone still measures weight, it is because it is good for business. Numbers are a very profitable proposition. Food, pharma, media – the weight loss industry feeds them all and feeds off them. In fact it casts its net much wider than these industries – why else do you think Google would buy Fitbit? Health, the way we perceive it, our obsession to track it with numbers, is a profitable proposition for many.

2. All-round vs one-dimensional approach to fitness

Once we move beyond weight loss, we discover that there are many aspects of a fit body – hormones, organs, bones, muscles, ligaments, tendons, joints, skin, hair and so much more. And that they don't work in isolation but are dependent on each other. It then becomes obvious that for the whole of us to stay healthy, a wholesome approach is necessary. One that accounts for all of the above and doesn't work in isolation on any one aspect. So no diets which come with a tag line – no exercise necessary, just walk; no exercise regime which says eat anything, just burn it all; no lifestyle which doesn't account for the need to sleep and recover. Food, activity, exercise and sleep together make for an all-round approach to sustainable health. And an all-round approach is necessary towards each of these aspects too – food not to be broken into carbs, proteins and fats; activity and exercise not to be restricted to walking or cardio; sleep and recovery on a daily basis and not weekend lie-ins.

Also, the daily constraints that life brings in, that is, your work, travel, family responsibilities, etc., have to become part of the solution and any diet or exercise pattern that doesn't account for them is bound not to succeed. Typical examples are of professions which require mental or physical effort through the day and their poor performance (low energy, migraines, missing periods, acidity, joint ache, etc.) on low-calorie diets like intermittent fasting, 2 meals a day, etc.

The biology of human starvation

As the Second World War ravaged Europe, the biggest killer was hunger. The entire population was starving and scientific information about the physiological effects of starvation was not available. Ancel Keys, a scientist in Minnesota, USA, considered the father of modern nutrition science, decided to conduct a study. In 1944 he recruited healthy adult volunteers for a yearlong experiment which was divided into three parts – the first three months to observe the regular eating pattern of the participants, the next six months of starvation and the last three months of rehabilitation. The most interesting point to note here is that to simulate starvation, participants were put on only two meals a day. This was to be accompanied with a regular daily routine and 6–7 kilometres of walking every day.

Within weeks of starving, participants reported a frightening decline in strength and energy levels. They felt old, constantly tired and irritable all the time. They suffered from 'mental apathy', wherein the everyday life, including sexual life, lost all relevance and they became obsessed with food. Their metabolism slowed down drastically and for many bowel movement reduced to once a week. Their blood volume reduced by 10%, there was swelling on the face, ankles and knees and their heart shrank in size. Most creepily, participants began to think everyone else looked too fat, rather than them looking too thin. Researchers later noted that this is the same mindset displayed by anorexics. On an average, they lost 25% of their body weight in those six months, even when they had not been overweight to begin with.

After the study was over, some participants reported eating as much as five times the quantity of food they normally ate. For years afterwards, they reported a constant sensation of hunger regardless of how much they ate. The study was published in 1951 as a landmark two-volume book, *The Biology of Human Starvation*.

The volunteers for this experiment did it for the sake of science and to help fellow human beings who were suffering from starvation. They described it as the worst time of their lives.

3. Long-term vs short-term solutions

The other aspect of sustainable health, one which is built into the meaning of the word sustainable, is the concept of long-term health. Every time you make a food choice or a decision to follow a certain diet trend or lifestyle, the first question you should ask yourself is – can I continue to do this for the rest of my life and am I happy even for my children to eat like this? If that sounds too much to comprehend, what about the next 15 years or even five years? If not, you should really rethink why you want to do this. Quick weight loss is not worth the long-term trouble it will bring along.

Although the human body is not designed to respond well to short-term measures, our brain, on the other hand, finds it very difficult to comprehend long term and is more interested in immediate rewards. This is what the weight loss industry uses to its benefit and the only way not to fall into that trap is to constantly remind yourself of this. Quick results, usually used as proxy for quick weight loss, can and mostly do lead to slow deterioration in the body, sometimes irreversible. We usually don't make the connection between that month-long liquid diet we did five years ago and the damage to the liver that shows up now.

The sensible route to good health

Health is a primary right, a human rights issue really. Even in a city like New York, Bronx would be poorer on health parameters than, say, Manhattan. Where we live, accessibility to health care, clean air and fresh produce and a multitude of other factors, including education, poverty and gender, affect our health. An interesting study in Newcastle, a charming university city in the UK, showed that people who lived in an area called Byke performed badly on health parameters compared to those who lived in Jesmond. Byke is a poor area, Jesmond a posh neighbourhood.

Closer to home, you have Delhi and Punjab ranking among the worst in health in India. A quick glance at their pollution levels tells you why. Your pin code is now emerging as a critical aspect in influencing your health. And this is irrespective of the country you live in. In cities, it's much more important as ghettos or poorer parts of any city bear the maximum burden of ill health.

On the other hand, the rich are sometimes led into believing that eating just two times will make them yogis or give them a 200% surge in growth hormone (kya karoge with all that GH, even if you actually get the surge) or eating only meat will turn them into a Maasai. 'Maasai dekha hai kya, Maasai?' asked my client. 'Khali meat khate hain woh log, so fit they are,' he informed me. Dekho boss, we are living in la la land if we feel that eating meat will make us like the Maasai – it won't. You drive around in your Mercedes, driver opens the door, EA carries your laptop, intern connects your VC even on a diet call. The Maasai roams freely in the jungle, can actually hunt or at least scare away the lion should there be an attack, lives in a hut and grazes the cows for miles (and doesn't count steps). You will not become a Maasai by eating meat – forget about it. Also, you are already 43, which makes you a very lucky Maasai because the average lifespan for Maasai men is about 42. (And let us not even go into the health struggles of the Maasai and the food insecurity they face.)

Keto or vegan?

Recently, there was a headline which declared that research has now proven that eating meat is not dangerous to health and that all these years we have been misled. They had looked at the same data that the studies which said limit meat intake had looked at and found their results to be statistically irrelevant. The keto community felt vindicated. On the other hand, the vegan community had lots to cheer about too. The documentary *Game Changers* was successfully converting the once hard-core meat eaters to plant-based diets. Virat Kohli even tweeted how he felt much better being a vegetarian athlete and that the diet he believed in all these years was a myth.

Almost on a daily basis, there are influencers who were once keto becoming vegan and dissing their earlier diets and vice versa. Where does that leave us commoners? In a pretty decent place, I would say. For starters, we must realize that food is as diverse as people are and it makes complete sense to eat the way we grew up eating. Without really complicating our lives, it provides us with nutrition and is cultural and climate-sensitive too.

It's really not about meat but eating it in a sustainable manner without it taking a toll on our body or the planet. So, if you are from a traditional meat-eating community, go back to the practice of eating meat sometimes, two to three times a week max and with rice or bhakri and sabzis, just like your grandmom taught you to. And if you are a vegetarian, don't worry about protein, just eat your dals and pulses with rice and bhakris and sabzis, just like your grandmom taught you to.

And if you want to go off dairy because of ill-treatment of cows, know that while that is true of industrial milk, it is not quite true for the majority of small farmers in India. We still have access (and inexpensive at that) to ethically sourced milk, why give that up for almond or soya milk? And then what about the land degradation and loss of ecology to produce almond milk for such a huge population?

So what is the answer then to keto or vegan? None of the above. Eat the way you grew up eating.

PS: All diet trends and food-related headlines are industry-backed.

At the end of the day, remember that the means to the end is much more important than the end in itself. At least, that is what yoga, Ayurveda and karma teaches us. For example, it's not about getting into that shirsasana but about how you get there. Do you get there with the strength in your core or with the fear of falling? Do you hastily plonk yourself up against the wall or teach the body to remain steady as the world goes upside down, even if it takes you a year to get there? You remember the story of the web the spider spun slowly and taught the lesson of a lifetime to the king even while saving him?

Let's take the example of shirsasana forward. Doing it the right way may cost you a year but then its impression will carry itself even into your next life. And during this life, it will teach you how to steady your spine when your Uber driver brakes abruptly, it will teach you how to lengthen your calves even as you strut around in your heels, it will make your digestion smoother, staying in the background and anchoring you through all this. It's the subconscious learning and the carry-over benefit to unrelated activities that more than justify the time it will take. The quick plonking up makes it look like you have got it but it comes with the constant fear of falling off and has no carry-over benefits.

In modern history, the only country where the population lost weight collectively (average of all adults) was Cuba. This was in the early 1990s, the Soviet Union had collapsed and the average calorie consumption of Cubans fell from 3000–3200 to about 2400. The US embargo led to food and fuel shortages and even public buses stopped running. Castro declared it a *periodo especial* (special period). The period saw food rationing, promotion of small-scale gardening and distribution of more than a million Chinese-made cycles. Not surprisingly, people lost weight (5.5 kg on average) and national averages for diabetes and heart disease dropped. The *British Medical Journal* covered this phenomenon, highlighting how eating less and moving more could be used as a population-based intervention.

But as the Cuban economy started picking up in the new millennium, obesity rates tripled from

1995 to 2011. Food and fuel were back, so were the rates of diabetes and heart disease. But ask any Cuban if they would like to go back to the 1990s and they will say they never ever want to go through that time of their life again. Even the authors who wrote about this in the *British Medical Journal* concluded that the 1990s tragedy was man-made (by international politics) and that it should never happen again to any population. They had high praise for the dignity and courage with which Cubans faced the social and economic challenges of the 'special period'.

Closer home, the people of Kashmir don't have access to the Internet for extended periods of time. If you did a population-based study, you could showcase how reduced screen time led to better health outcomes, decrease in tech-neck posture and lower-back aches and improved quality of sleep. But once restrictions are lifted no Kashmiri would pine for or romanticize the Internet blockage that reduced screen time. They would go back with a vengeance to the gadgets.

Long story short, the only way to improve health without an economic or security crisis is to take the more sensible and sustainable route towards it – education, advocacy, self-regulation. This forms the foundation of the fitness project too – you have to own the guidelines and work towards them one day at a time, no ghai. Be the tortoise, not the hare. It's not about losing weight, it's about doing it the right, sustainable way. Come, turn the page and let's start.

Chapter 3

The 12 guidelines

The 12 guidelines can be divided into the following three categories:

1. Food and eating practices based – these guidelines ask you to include local and culturally compliant foods and follow time-tested eating practices. Along with following the guidelines, you can practise the 3 S's of eating right – sit, silence and senses. Whenever possible, sit down in sukhasana to eat your meals, eat in silence and use your hands to eat.

2. Physical activity and exercise based – these guidelines urge you to engineer movement into your daily life and also to do regular exercise. They emphasize the difference between activity and exercise and explain how

both are crucial for good health.

3. Daily habits based – these guidelines focus on the harmful effect of gadgets, especially on sleep and recovery, and also provide ideas to reduce the contact of plastic with your food and water on a daily basis.

Before we start with the guidelines, a short note on how best to implement them in your daily life.

1. Following the guidelines

The best way to follow the guidelines of the 12-week project is in a cumulative manner. This means, in week 2, you follow week 1 + week 2 guidelines, in week 3 you follow week 1 + week 2 + week 3 guidelines, and so on. This process is easier and allows you to slowly transition into a sustainable lifestyle. It's also tried and tested and worked beautifully for all the participants of the project.

You may be tempted to start following all 12 guidelines at one go from week 1, but that can be very challenging. The whole idea is to make these habits long-lasting.

2. Customizing the advice

The guidelines are generic in nature. You will have to fine-tune or tweak the advice. This will depend on many factors like your food likes/dislikes, where you live, season and climate, your work hours, family commitments, practicality, etc. Wherever possible, multiple options are given in the guidelines and you can choose what works best for you. Also, note that the food-related guidelines don't specify the recipe or details of preparation of the food items and you are expected to use time-tested recipes and preparations from your household.

3. **Weekly compliance**

If for some reason you have not been able to follow the guidelines in a particular week, don't stress – take it easy and continue with the process from next week onward. Even during the project, we asked the participants to note down their weekly compliance as follows – mostly, 50–50, not really. Even those who noted down '50–50' or 'not really' for some weeks but continued the programme at their own pace saw a huge improvement in their health.

4. **Measuring progress**

You can measure your progress as follows:

(a) How well you are doing on your health parameters on a scale of 1–5, where higher rating means you are doing better.

Parameters to measure – energy levels during the day, sleep quality at night, acidity/

bloating/indigestion, sweet cravings after meals, compliance with exercise, pain during PMS/period (for women).

(b) Inch loss at waist. Measure it at the navel. You can also measure waist to hip ratio. This is the waist circumference at navel divided by hip circumference (your hip measurement is taken at the widest point in your hips).

(c) Home fitness tests to measure strength, flexibility, stamina. You can easily find instructions online for these tests. The most popular home fitness tests are:
  - Sit and reach
  - Plank hold
  - Step test
  - Wall sit test

(d) You can also measure the progress on the following parameters – HbA1C, HDL, TSH, vitamin D, vitamin B12

Measure your progress at four points of time:
- Before starting with the guidelines
- One month after starting
- Two months after starting
- Three months after starting

Week 1

Guideline

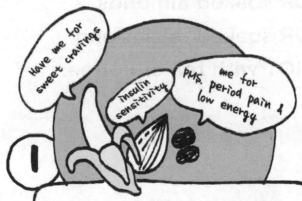

Start your day with a Banana or any fresh fruit OR soaked almonds OR soaked raisins and NOT with tea or coffee.

The Guideline

Start your day with
a banana or any fresh fruit
OR soaked almonds
OR soaked raisins and
NOT with tea or coffee.

Notes

★ It's okay to have chai or coffee 10–15 minutes after this meal

★ Have a glass of (only) plain water and then have this meal

★ Eat this within 20 minutes of waking up or after the thyroid pill if you are on one

★ You can work out, do yoga, etc., 15–20 minutes after having the banana/almonds/raisins

★ If not working out, you can have your breakfast within an hour of this meal

★ Don't add anything to the water you are having in the morning – just have plain water

★ You can drink the water in which you have soaked the raisins

★ You can also add 1–2 strands of kesar when soaking the raisins

Why?

☑ Banana: For all those who have digestion issues or get sugar cravings after a meal. Buy fresh, local variety. Buy at least 2 to 3 times a week and do not bring them home in plastic bags – use a cloth bag instead.

☑ 7–8 soaked raisins with 1–2 strands of kesar – if you have rated yourself as a person with terrible PMS or with low energy through the day.

☑ 4–6 soaked and peeled badam – if you have insulin resistance, diabetes, PCOD or low fertility or poor sleep quality. Pick the mamra or the local variety of badam – it's richer in nutrients. For PCOD, switch to 7–8 raisins and 1–2 strands of kesar 10 days before periods.

Raisins and kesar for PMS

Raisins are known to reduce acidity, constipation and bloating. This knowledge is part of our indigenous wisdom, stuff that is accessible to all and bastion of none. Just like how we know the benefits of haldi or tulsi or sonth (dry ginger). Kesar too is known for its many benefits, including its ability to improve skin tone and boost fertility levels. Through the fitness project we made a conscious attempt to dip into our oral wisdom and use it to prevent/heal modern ailments.

The combination of raisins and kesar first thing in the morning was probably our most successful guideline. Women who'd had bad or painful periods for years reported a drop in anxiety, cramps and acidity within weeks; many of them even experienced totally pain-free periods for the first time in their lives.

It could be the iron, magnesium, B6 or fibre of the raisins or even the combination of these with the volatile oils of kesar, but the magic was in its consistent use. Small quantities but for days together. It also helped reduce sweet cravings later in the day.

FAQs

Q. I don't like banana, what should I do?

A. Pick any regional, local fruit that is currently in season.

Q. I have a bit of all three issues, what should I eat now – banana or almonds or raisins?

A. Pick the one you most like eating as the first meal in the morning. Also, feel free to eat banana today, almonds tomorrow, raisins day after. Essentially, learn to be self-dependent, that's the name of the game, buddy.

Q. So if I am PCOD, what exactly should I eat?

A. Soaked almonds and then 10 days before periods switch to soaked raisins and kesar. If you are unable to predict period date, make the switch when you begin to feel bloated or irritated. This can be followed for endometriosis and adenomyosis too.

Q. Why are we soaking the almonds?

A. To unlock the nutrients from it and to allow the phytic acid levels (which can otherwise bind to minerals like zinc and make them unavailable for our body) to go down.

Remember that fitness is built one step at a time by small but daily actions. The body rewards consistency over anything else. And consistently having your first meal within 15 minutes of waking up is a big step forward.

Week 2

Guideline

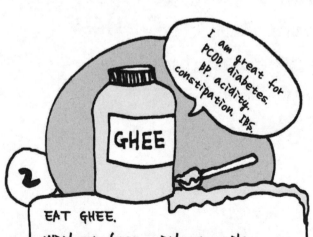

I am great for PCOD, diabetes, BP, acidity, constipation, IBS.

2

EAT GHEE.
without fear. without guilt.
without doubt. Add 1 tsp of ghee
to breakfast. lunch and dinner

The Guideline

Eat ghee. Without fear,
without guilt, without
doubt. Add 1 tsp of ghee
to breakfast, lunch and
dinner.

Notes

From the shastras to your nanis and dadis and now even the *Sunday Mail* of London and Cleveland Clinic of USA, everyone sings its glories. It keeps you company from birth to death, in sickness and in health and through the good and the bad. It has been maligned by the food and the weight loss industry for the longest time and demonized even by the medical and the pharma industry, but satya aur ghee ki hamesha jeet hoti hai.

★ You can have your breakfast 20–90 minutes after the first meal that you have been having from week 1.
★ Add an extra tsp of ghee to lunch if you have sweet cravings or experience an afternoon slump where you feel that you are operating on 50% potential.
★ Add an extra tsp of ghee to dinner if you wake up feeling constipated, have irritable bowel syndrome or digestion issues in general or suffer from poor sleep quality.

★ Here are some other ways in which you can consume ghee, especially in winter, to keep the joints supple and skin glowing:

- Have ghee-roasted makhanas as a mid-meal around chai time, say, 4 p.m.
- Have gond laddoos made in ghee, especially if you live in North India or in parts of the world with harsh winters, as a mid-morning meal, 2–3 hours after breakfast.
- Have ghee and jaggery after lunch or dinner if you suffer from PMS, fatigue or low haemoglobin (Hb) levels.

Why?

☑ Ghee by nature is lipolytic, that is, it's a fat that breaks down other fats. This is good as it mobilizes fats from stubborn fat areas of the body.

☑ Ghee helps you de-stress, sleep better and wake up fresher – as it allows for better digestion, assimilation of nutrients and eases bowel movement.

☑ Rich in antioxidants, conjugated linoleic acid (CLA) and fat soluble vitamins like A, E, D, ghee has just what you need for a healthy heart. Especially useful for PCOD, diabetes and heart diseases, BP, acidity, weak joints, constipation, IBS.

☑ Addition of ghee to meals reduces their glycaemic index and helps regulate blood sugar.

FAQs

Q: I have cholesterol/high triglycerides/ fatty liver/BP issues. Can I have ghee?

A: Yes, totally. Ghee regulates cholesterol by increasing the contribution of lipids towards metabolism. Cut back on packaged products like biscuits and avoid alcohol, not ghee. Ghee is safe.

Q: I am overweight/have diabetes/ PCOD. Can I have ghee?

A: Yes, essential fatty acids like the one found in ghee help accelerate fat loss and help regulate blood sugar (reduce risk of obesity-related diseases).

Q: We cook in ghee, do we need to add an extra tsp on top of that?

A: That's your choice. Ensure that you are getting 3–6 tsp of ghee per day per person. The key is that ghee should enhance the flavour of food and not mask it.

Q: We cook in oil, can we add ghee on top before eating?

A: Yes, you should add ghee.

Q: Is the store-bought ghee okay if we can't make it at home?

A: Yes, but then check that it is from desi cow milk. Patronize ghee from small gaushalas and small women cooperatives over large corporations.

Q: If desi cow ghee is not available, can we make from buffalo milk?

A: Yes, you can. This is better than buying ghee from big brands.

Q: Options for those outside India?

A: Cultured white organic butter or clarified butter that is sold in health food stores. Look for free grazing, grass-fed cow milk products.

Q: Do I need to add ghee to non-veg food also? Doesn't it already have fat?

A: Yes, you should. The unique fatty acid structure of ghee is very helpful for the body.

Q: How do we know how much ghee is to be added in each meal?

A: It depends on what you are eating and this info is part of our collective food wisdom. Foods like dal–rice, khichdi, roti–sabzi will require less ghee

52

compared to puran poli, dal–baati, bajra (pearl millet) roti, etc. Ask your grandmother if you have any confusion.

Q: I don't like ghee. What are my options?

A: To develop a taste for ghee is one option but, jokes apart, make a conscious effort to include nuts, coconut and kache ghani ka or cold pressed groundnut/mustard/til/coconut oil (depending on the region you come from) in your diet. You can even start eating the regular peanut or curry patta or mulgapodi mixed with til or gingelly oil to make up for ghee in your diet.

Things we don't know or don't bother to know about ghee

- Ghee has antibacterial and antiviral properties. Other than helping you recover from sickness, it ensures that you don't fall sick.
- The antioxidants in ghee make it the miraculous anti-wrinkling and anti-ageing therapy you were searching for.
- Ghee is excellent for joint health as it lubricates and oxygenates them.
- Ghee takes nutrients from your food and delivers them through fat-permeable membranes like in the brain.
- Ghee regulates your satiety signal and ensures you eat the right amount of food.

Week 3

Guideline

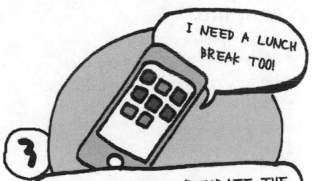

I NEED A LUNCH BREAK TOO!

RETHINK, REFORM & REGULATE THE USE OF GADGETS IN YOUR LIFE.

No gadgets during meals
- start with one main meal.
No gadgets atleast 30 to 60 mins before sleeping.

The Guideline

Rethink, reform, and regulate the use of gadgets in your life.

- At least one meal without gadgets
- No gadget 30 minutes before sleeping
- Keep phone at eye level when using it

Notes

Well, all talk about fitness is useless if it doesn't make you rethink the way you are living your life. It's about paying attention to little things that matter and not just about talking and googling carbs, protein, fat and calories.

So, from this week, you will take the first step to developing a strong back, flat stomach and a tall stance. This is what I want you to do.

★ When eating meals, no gadgets. Start doing this at one meal a day and over the next 10 weeks, build it to all three main meals. Decide which meal you will start this from – breakfast, lunch or dinner.

★ Before going to bed, no gadgets for 30 minutes. So don't delay bedtime, just keep the phone away, switch off your TV and read a book (not on Kindle or iPad).

★ When you do use the phone in the day, check for your posture. The correct way is to lift the phone to eye level and not tilt the neck down.

One of the things this will do is limit your phone usage to only the relevant and important issues as raising the phone doesn't make for a good picture.

I know this is a tough one, but it's worth doing. 'Sar utha ke jiyo' should be your motto now.

Why?

☑ We are more attuned to our hunger signals when we are paying full attention to what we are eating. Eating in a distracted manner is a sure-shot way to overeat.

☑ The brain interprets light emitted by gadgets as daylight and doesn't allow the hormonal shift to night-time. This leads to poor sleep and recovery during the night and lethargy during the day.

☑ The human head is heavy and we have spent months as babies learning to stabilize it. In a neutral position, ears above the shoulders, the head weighs 5–6 kg. But with just a 15-degree tilt downwards it weighs more than double, about 15 kg; at 30 degrees it's 20 kg; and at 60 degrees it's as much as 30 kg. What do you think this is doing to your back, shoulders and even to the brain? Most of us want to lose fat from our stomachs, sport flatter abs and have a narrower waist, but it's impossible with all that slouching and so-called technology posture, which is that much more harmful for people dealing with diabetes, heart problems and other hormonal issues like PCOD and thyroid. It even interferes with the proper functioning of our adrenal glands and hampers cardiorespiratory processes.

FAQs

Q: I need to be accessible at all times, how can I cut down on my phone usage?

A: Well, in that case, chin up and take it as an occupational hazard but be aware of the risks it brings you. And then work harder to cut down on mindless scrolling and surfing on the phone. Essentially, just rethink your phone usage. Do you really need to open the good morning GIF, autoplay videos or send that eye roll emoticon to everyone you talk to?

Q: Is there really anything that links health hazards to gadget usage?

A: Yes, there is plenty. But industry influence on policy-making is so deeply entrenched that it is difficult if not completely impossible to 'prove' the health hazards. We all know how long it took before the cigarette industry allowed the 'injurious to health' warning to go on its packaging and how they continue to fight tooth and nail for the size of the warning. But the very fact that phones themselves now allow you to track your screen time, put alerts that notify you that you have been online for too long, etc., should tell you that there is much more truth to the health hazards than what makes it to the press. There is also a Padma Shri doctor who is trying to lobby with the Government of India to put injurious to health warnings on gadgets. Then there is Instagram, which is experimenting with not letting the number of likes show up on your page. The proof as they say is in the pudding.

Q: But I use my phone as an alarm.

A: Just get yourself a real alarm clock, it will even look nice on your bedside table and it will be charming to wake up to a ghanti that you can't put on snooze.

Week 4

Guideline

Remember me as the mouth of the clock! I want a wholesome meal not a snack!

Eat a wholesome meal between 4-6 pm in the evening. Plan for it in advance. Some options - handful of nuts. Poha. Upma. Dosa. Egg toast. homemade khakra...

The Guideline

Eat a wholesome meal between 4 and 6 p.m.

Notes

I always tell my clients that the key to them losing weight lies in what they eat between 4 and 6 p.m., a time when most of us are the most hungry and also the most careless in our eating. For me, this is the single most important meal of the day.

Also, you must have heard this: have a light dinner to lose weight. But how to make dinner light? Well, by eating something wholesome in the evening. This is the make-or-break meal, this decides whether you will have long-lasting fitness or whether your resolve will fizzle out in the next couple of weeks.

Depending on when you eat dinner, the 4 to 6 p.m. meal can be relatively light or heavy, but it should always be wholesome. Some meal options whether you are at work, on a train, in college, wherever:

★ Handful of groundnuts and chana. This regulates appetite, prevents bloating and overeating at dinner-time. Do this if you eat dinner early, before 8 p.m. Very good meal for diabetics, for PCOD and those with low energy levels in the day.

★ Jaggery, ghee and chapatti. If you stay active, work away from home, eat dinner after 9 p.m. and struggle to sleep well, suffer from constipation or have low Hb levels.

★ Poha/upma/dosa/egg toast/homemade khakra or mathri/homemade gond or besan laddoo. If your workload increases after 6 p.m. or you have a party to attend or if you have frequent headaches, leg cramps, low immunity, this is a good meal. And if none of the above is possible, even a grilled vegetable and cheese sandwich, Mumbai ishtyle.

★ Chaat/samosa/street food. Yes and this is a good time to have it, but only once a week. And the worst time to have chaat or street food is dinner-time.

In all cases, expect dinner quantity to naturally drop over the next four to five days. This is normal and an expected outcome.

The trick to getting this right is to plan this in advance. Plan for your whole week today.

Why?

☑ The hormone cortisol follows a natural cycle. It rises in the morning, allowing you to start fresh, clear bowels, etc., and drops in the evening, to allow for restful sleep at night. That is why waking up fresh and quality of sleep are health parameters we are tracking in this project. Because this tells us about your metabolic health, your immune response, your hormonal balance and your response to stress.

☑ When we don't eat anything in the evening or kill our appetite with chai or coffee, our body works at producing more cortisol instead of reducing it. This will lead to:
- Overeating at dinner
- Poor sleep
- Slow digestion
- PCOD/thyroid issues
- Insulin insensitivity (leading to diabetes and many other lifestyle diseases)

More meal options for 4–6 p.m.

Meal options	Most useful when/for	Additional notes
• Handful of peanuts and chana • Makhana roasted in ghee with rock salt • Fresh seasonal fruit or banana • Chikki • Homemade chakli or muruku	• If dinner is by 7 or 7.30 p.m. • Insulin resistance and PCOD • Diabetes or BP	• Goes best with early risers, exercisers and sleepers
• Roti with ghee and jaggery • Dahi rice, jhalmoori • Idli podi ghee	• If dinner is after 9 p.m. • Longer than 90 minutes travel from office to work • If Hb levels are low	• Helps improve sleep quality • Relieves constipation • Improves energy levels
• Poha, upma • Homemade thepla or mathri with pickle • Homemade khakra with jeeradu and ghee • Homemade dosa • Gond/besan/ nariyal-rava laddoo • Egg toast • Protein shake	• If workload increases in the evening • You have a party to go to • You make good food at home but don't know when to eat • If dinners are erratic • If you routinely work late into the night	• Beats mood swings and midnight cravings • Boosts immunity • Prevents lethargy and leg cramps and weakness

FAQs

Q: If you have very early dinner, like at 6.30–7 p.m.?

A: You must be having your lunch early and the 4–6 p.m. snack in your case can be had between 3 and 5 p.m. You can choose one of the lighter options from the list on p. 69.

Q: If you work out in the evening?

A: Have your 4 R's post workout (rehydrate with water, replenish glycogen stores, repair with protein and recover with antioxidants – details in my book *Don't Lose Out, Work Out*), including a banana and a protein shake and this becomes your wholesome meal. If you work out at about 7 p.m., you can have any of the above meal options latest by 5.30 p.m. and your dinner immediately after the workout.

Q: For night shift or odd working hours?

A: You just have to move the timing accordingly. Your 4–6 p.m. meal could be earlier or later according to your working hours.

4. What not to have at this time?

A: The 4–6 p.m. meal needs to be wholesome. This means no oil-free, sugar-free, exotic fruits, juices or any 'diet' options. Have a traditional meal the way it is supposed to be. You will lose all the benefits of this meal if you mess up the basics. As much as possible, stick to the easy and made-at-home options listed on p. 69.

Week 5

Guideline

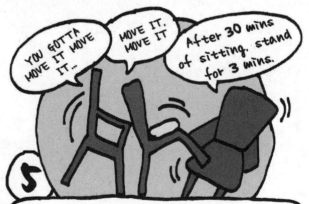

The Guideline

Move more, sit less.

- For every 30 minutes of sitting, stand up for 3 minutes
- Take the stairs at home and work, every day
- Once a week, do a task currently assigned to paid help or a gadget
- Take 100 easy steps after dinner

Notes

Through these guidelines, I have been trying to highlight the obvious but often overlooked aspects of health and fitness. And this week it's about something even more basic than exercise – activity. Because without an active lifestyle, exercise can bring you no benefits.

The problem in our world today is that we sit too much. We are much more sedentary than we ever were. We sit on trains, in cars, in offices, while watching TV, talking on the phone, playing video games, you name it. We are an inactive community, especially all of us in urban and semi-urban settings, and it's time to change.

Sitting is now identified as an independent risk factor for lifestyle diseases, much like smoking. It means that even if you are eating right, working out, sleeping on time, not stressed, etc., but sit too much, you are still at risk of lifestyle diseases and even death.

A study done way back in 1949 on London bus drivers and conductors revealed that drivers were much more prone to heart diseases and stroke compared to conductors. On an average a conductor would take 500–700 steps more per working day. So they lived longer and stayed healthier. Essentially it boils down to basics – human beings were meant for constant activity and not constant sitting.

Here are some easy ways to move more, sit less:

★ For every 30 minutes of sitting, stand for at least 3 minutes

★ When you stand, stand with your weight well distributed on both feet

★ Take the stairs at work or home, every day. At least climb four floors every day.

★ Park your car as far as possible, keep at least 500 steps between your car and your destination. Paris by the way is banning cars from the city by 2030.

★ Once every week, walk around your neighbourhood or walk your child to school or park, friend's house, restaurant, etc. Walking is good not just as an activity, but also at building strong community bonds and for the environment.

★ Once every week, do at least one task that is currently being done by house help or a gadget – wash your own clothes, do dishes for the entire household, sweep and swab your house.

★ Men are not exempt! You can cook a meal and/ or clean up after the family has eaten at least once a week. You can make just dal–rice or khichdi but building a nurturing environment is crucial for good health too.

★ 100 steps or shatapavli after dinner. It's a rough measure, where you walk, more like stroll for 5–10 minutes. Even if you just clear the table and clean the kitchen post a meal, it would meet the requirements of shatapavli.

You may not realize the importance of movement and activity but it maintains brain plasticity, especially in older adults, and also helps prevent back pain, diabetes, heart disease and even depression. Move now, leave sitting for the lesser and later.

And remember, activity is different from exercise, and is not a substitute. We will discuss exercise in detail in coming guidelines.

FAQs

Q: A lot of my work is done sitting.

A: Take breaks as often as you can, stand as often as you can and walk to the people you need to chat with instead of using the office messenger or WhatsApp. Walk and talk, just without the phone;) Also, consider buying yourself a footrest, so that you can rest your feet and allow for the back of the knee to open out and receive better blood circulation.

Q: What about long meetings?

A: Consider using the huddle table – people get to the agenda quickly, discuss and disperse. The conventional conference room is not just about endless sitting but also eating mindlessly – little wonder that it makes for such a tiring combo.

Q: Come on, I still need to sit.

A: Yes, do so by all means. Even my work involves sitting and here's what I have done to help myself. Bought myself a bench instead of a chair and I sit cross-legged on it, instead of having my feet dangling. The key is to be aware of the dangers of long sitting hours and taking small but sensible steps to reduce it.

Week 6

Guideline

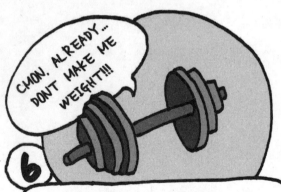

Start with at least one session of strength training every week. IF never done before, start once a week with beginners routine from Dont lose out workout.

The Guideline

Start with at least one session of strength training every week.

Notes on strength/weight training

This week's guideline is a straight call from the heart – exercise. You know you should be doing it but you are still looking for a good time. Good time aa gaya.

There isn't a person on earth who doesn't want to lose weight but to lose weight you have to gain weight – lean body weight – the weight of your bones and muscles.

Most of us lose 2–4 kilos of muscles every 10 years. In women, especially after 30, we lose muscle from our thighs and gain intramuscular fat at a fast pace. This continuous and progressive loss of muscle and bone density can be reversed with exercise. Not just exercise actually, but structured exercise. One that includes strength (weight) training and follows some basic principles of exercise science.

★ **If you have never weight trained before:**
Start now. Schedule a meeting with an expert trainer at a local gym and begin with a once-

a-week routine. You can also use the beginner's routine from *Don't Lose Out, Work Out*. You must start especially if you already have insulin resistance, are very obese, have a heart condition, bone loss or diabetes. That much more important for older adults (men and women).

★ **If you are already training but are not regular:** Get regular and dedicate at least two times a week to strength training. This is especially crucial for all those who have PCOD or breakouts, are menopausal or have thyroid issues. Focus on bringing in progressive overload into your workouts. Read more about it in the 'Strength Training' chapter in *Don't Lose Out, Work Out* and follow the intermediate routine.

★ **If you are training three or more days a week** Shabash! Drop your reps to 5–8 and focus on the intensity or the actual weight you subject your muscles to (advanced routine from *Don't Lose Out, Work Out*). The biggest gains of strength training come from the load bearing that you train your muscles to do.

Why?

As we get older, our fat begins to infiltrate even our muscles, and our anabolic response, or how well we respond to exercise, begins to drop. And strength training is a good intervention to turn that around. It uses up extra fat stores, enlarges your muscle size and strength and ensures density of bones and lubrication of joints. Strength training is extremely effective but an undervalued intervention for maintaining hormonal health. It keeps your insulin sensitive and stimulates growth hormone. Here are some more advantages:

- ☑ Prevents diabetes and if you already have it, strength training has the potential to get you on lower dosages if not totally off medicines

- ☑ Regulates period cycle and leads to pain-free periods. Makes conception easy if you want a baby.

- ☑ Reduces arthritic pain and uric acid

- ☑ Reduces blood pressure and resting heart rate

☑ Improves functioning of the brain

☑ Increases gait speed (can walk faster)

☑ Reduces depressive thoughts and improves sleep

List endless hai, boss, but the thing is that all of us talk about how we gain weight post 30, but we are losing muscle, so then what weight are we gaining? That of fat. The tissue that doesn't add to your mobility, strength, agility or sex appeal. But you cannot measure fatness on the weighing scale. So get off the weighing scale and get under a squat rack.

FAQs

Q: I already do cardio/swimming/zumba/ dancing, etc., should I strength train?

A: Yes. And the reason is afterburn or excessive post-exercise oxygen consumption (EPOC). Afterburn is a process that follows every session of strength training, where the body burns fat at a higher rate for up to 36–48 hours. This is not the case with aerobic exercises, where fat burn, if at all, happens only during the duration of exercise.

This is especially helpful for the obese or those suffering from hormonal imbalances due to excessive body fat.

Q: Is there an alternative to gym that we can do at home?

A: The thing is that you can train at home. It's not as effective as training in the gym but it is infinitely better than not strength training at all. Squats, lunges and modified push-ups/pull-ups can be safely done at home. This link has some good home exercises: http://www.exrx.net/Questions/ BasicProgram.html

Two scenarios:

1. You have access but don't want to go to the gym because you are apprehensive/shy/don't have time/it's too loud/it's for bodybuilders only, etc.

   The benefits of weight training outweigh all of the above concerns. Working out in a gym is the safest way to weight train as you can use machines and light weights (lighter than body weight) to train with a proper form. By gradually increasing weight, you can make progress in your strength.

2. You don't have access to a gym at all.

   In that case, you can learn some basic strengthening exercises that use minimum or no equipment.

Q: I have just started weight training, my blood sugar levels are better, my thyroid is better, my jeans are getting loose, but I haven't lost a gram, in fact I have GAINED a couple of kilos! :(

A: First things first, change that sad face to a broadly smiling one. Weight training increases fat-free weight, that of your bones and muscles. Obviously, that's going to mean some additional grams or kilos to your body mass. Not to forget the fact that as you start storing more muscle glycogen, it adds to body weight too.

Technically you can gain or lose up to 5 kilos of body weight without gaining or losing a single gram of fat. Body weight is no measure of fatness or fitness. Look at exercise performance instead – it's the sure-shot measure of your body's fat-burning ability (health, fitness and risk of diseases). If you are pushing more weight, feeling more enthusiastic about exercise, looking forward to your routine in the gym, it means you are on track. That's it.

Rules for exercise planning

✓ Plan for at least 150 minutes of total workout time in the week

✓ Keep at least a 2-day gap between two weight training sessions

✓ If doing cardio also, schedule it a day after weight training

✓ Build in rest days to get the best out of exercise days

✓ Yoga asanas are an excellent form of both exercise and recovery (and much more). And can be done daily.

ABOUT ALL EXERCISE

It's not just important but crucial that we exercise

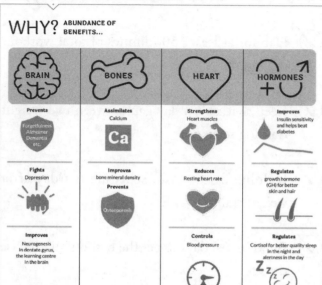

WHY? ABUNDANCE OF BENEFITS...

BRAIN	BONES	HEART	HORMONES
Prevents Forgetfulness Alzheimer Dementia etc.	**Assimilates** Calcium **Ca**	**Strengthens** Heart muscles	**Improves** Insulin sensitivity and helps beat diabetes
Fights Depression	**Improves** bone mineral density **Prevents** Osteoporosis	**Reduces** Resting heart rate	**Regulates** growth hormone (GH) for better skin and hair
Improves Neurogenesis in dentate gyrus, the learning centre in the brain		**Controls** Blood pressure	**Regulates** Cortisol for better quality sleep in the night and alertness in the day

HOW? BY FOLLOWING A PROPER STRUCTURE

RULES FOR EXERCISE PLANNING

Keep atleast a 2 day gap between two weight training sessions	Schedule cardio a day after weight training	Build in recovery days to get the best out of exercise days	Yoga asanas are an excellent form of exercise, recovery and much more (And can be done daily)	Plan for at least 150 mins of total workout time in the week

WEEKLY EXERCISE CALENDAR*

*You can modify depending on your current exercise routine

DAY 1	DAY 2	DAY 3	DAY 4	DAY 5	DAY 6	DAY 7
Weight training	40 mins CARDIO Easy run/ swim/ cycling/ dance	Active rest/ Yoga asana	Weight training	Yoga asana/ Hobby	20 mins SPEED WORKOUTS Sprints/ jumps, etc.	Active rest

WHAT TO EAT? EATING RIGHT IS CRUCIAL TO ENSURE THAT EXERCISE WORKS FOR YOU

Pre-workout meal

4 R's of Post workout meal

Pre-workout meal	Rehydrate	Replenish	Repair	Recover
Have a fruit 15-20 mins before a workout or a main meal 60-90 mins before	Drink enough water to quench your thirst and then have some more	Replenish the glycogen stores with a fruit like banana	Drink a whey protein shake to help in the repair processes	Have antioxidants like Vit C, Vit E, Selenium, Zinc, etc. for quick recovery

TOP 5 FOODS TO IMPROVE EXERCISE PERFORMANCE

Hand pounded
Keeps the gut strong
Good source of BCAA
(branch chain amino acids)

Easy to digest
Local
Prebiotic
Single polished
Avoid brown rice

RICE

Rich in minerals
Sweet potato
Sabudana Arbi Rich in fibre
Good for women

TUBERS
Suran
Rich in vitamins

Keeps our hormones balanced
For skin glow

Rich in folic acid

Indian superfood

ALIV
Rich in iron

Garden Cress Seeds

Right ratio of essential to non essential amino acids

WHEY PROTEIN
Speed up your recovery

Useful for the older adults who are exercising routinely

Easy on the stomach

Strong fat burner
Wholesome meal
Consume tender, ripe, dry and the water

COCONUT
Regulates blood pressure
Strong immunity

Week 7

Guideline

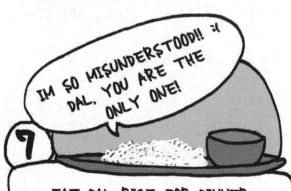

IM SO MISUNDERSTOOD!! :(
DAL, YOU ARE THE
ONLY ONE!

7

EAT DAL RICE FOR DINNER.
Cook it the way your grandmom
did. Eat white. not brown. Must
add ghee.

The Guideline

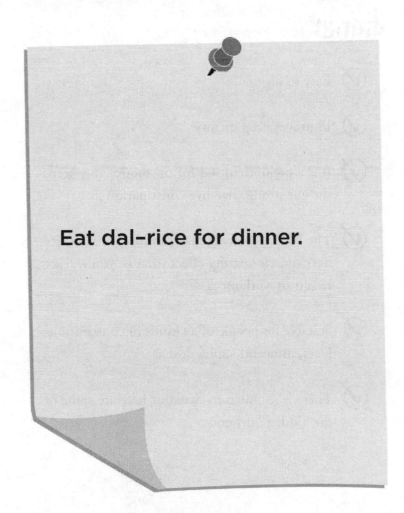

Eat dal-rice for dinner.

Why you should eat rice for dinner

✓ Easy to digest

✓ Improves sleep quality

✓ It is a prebiotic (food for probiotic) and keeps the gut strong. Bye-bye constipation.

✓ The BCAA (branch chain amino acids) in rice have muscle-sparing effect (that is, you will see results of workout faster)

✓ Suitable for people of all kinds of constitutions (vata, pitta and kapha doshas)

✓ There is so much to rice, but here are some of the hidden nutrients:

- Methionine – it's a sulphur-containing amino acid that helps prevent damage to the skin tone by free radicals, helps detox the liver and slows down the ageing process. Better skin and hair, fewer lines and less greying.
- Vitamin B1 – good for the nerves and heart and helps reduce inflammation and bloating. Also a good source of B3. You can increase values if you soak rice for a while before cooking it.
- RS – resistant starch, a molecule that gets fermented in our large intestines. It helps prevent cancer, improves lipid profile and inhibits of the growth bad bacteria.

Who can eat rice?

Everyone. The way we Indians eat rice, with dal and ghee, ensures that the meal stays low on the glycaemic index and there is a steady blood sugar response. It is therefore perfectly fine for anyone with diabetes, heart disease or any other disease, for pregnant women, for young and old, active and sedentary, thin and obese. In fact, a recent study presented at the European Congress of Obesity in Glasgow observed that though low-carb diets were popular in the West, addition of rice to one's diet could help reduce worldwide prevalence of obesity by 1% or about 7 million less obese people. The fibre, nutrients and plant compounds found in rice are associated with an increase in a feeling of fullness and therefore reduction in risks of overeating.

Rice is good for all 12 months but don't forget millets like jowar, bajra, ragi or even kuttu, rajgeera, samo, etc., which are eaten during fasts or on special occasions. You can have one of the millets or even wheat chapatti for one meal and rice for the other. You can even have rice for all three meals but ensure that you eat millets too.

FAQs

Q: How to cook rice?

A: Cook it the way in which it tastes the best, which is invariably how your grandmother used to. There is no such thing as 'removing starch' from rice; starch is an essential nutrient, along the molecules of which many other nutrients reside. 'Removing water' from rice removes these anti-ageing nutrients too. And if at all it is removed, traditionally, it would be cooked along with some grains and offered as kanji or pej to the oldest and the youngest members of the family as it's easy on the gastrointestinal tract, is liquid so no need to chew much (and you may either have not grown your teeth or lost your teeth) and the vitamin B helps in metabolic processes. So the removal of water came out of more intelligent use of resources and not from fear of getting fat. Eating rice at night is a brilliant strategy for those who plan to but don't work out in the morning, as it can really help with restorative sleep.

Q: Brown or white rice?

A: Hand-pounded or single-polished white rice.

Too much fibre in brown rice comes in the way of absorption of minerals like zinc, crucial for insulin function.

Q: Which rice to eat?

A: There are thousands of varieties of rice in India, each one having its own distinct aroma and flavour. These aromatic compounds provide many nutritional benefits and work like antioxidants in the body, helping defy the effects of ageing. So eat the variety that grows in (or closest to) the region you live in.

Q: Rice and roti together?

A: Yes, you can if you have the appetite.

Q: What if we have late dinner? Can we still have rice?

A: Yes, it's the easiest meal to digest. You can have it as khichdi or dal–rice.

Q: Can diabetics have rice?

A: Rice is traditionally eaten with dal/sabzi/meat/dahi, etc., along with ghee, and this lowers the glycaemic index of meals and is therefore totally safe for diabetics.

Q: I feel hungry later if I have only dal–rice?

A: Make sure you add ghee to your dal–rice and eat slowly and with full attention. Have a glass of milk before sleeping if still hungry.

Q: How much?

A: If you are having a wholesome meal between 4 and 6 p.m. and are exercising and keeping gadgets away during mealtimes, you will be eating just right. Nothing more, nothing less. More about quantity in the next guideline.

Week 8

Guideline

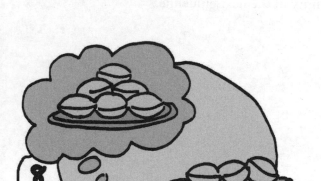

Use the mental meal map to help you eat the right quantity. Visualize how much would you like to eat. Serve yourself half of that portion. Take double the time to eat the meal.

The Guideline

Use the mental meal map as a tool to help you eat the right quantity.

Notes

When the eyes become clear, body healthy and appetite increases, it's a sign of success, according to the *Hatha Yoga Pradipika*. No wonder then that when you portion control, force yourself to eat less, mask your appetite with tea/coffee/chewing gum/soups/fibre gels, etc., success, even on the path of weight loss, becomes elusive.

A good life is where you are able to tell the difference between your need and greed. A life where you learn to enjoy food, fitness and health without feelings of guilt, remorse and frustration. But today we feel that we are fat because we eat too much or consume too many calories. The truth is that we live in 'obesogenic environments' – we have created situations and formed habits where it's almost impossible for us to nurture our appetite and eat just the right amount. And so, we have the mental meal map, a simple tool that anyone can use to understand their appetite and learn how much to eat.

The infographic below explains the simple steps of the mental meal map.

Step 1: Visualize how much you would like to eat
Step 2: Serve yourself half of that portion
Step 3: Take double time to eat this meal
       (or the same time as your full portion)
Step 4: If still hungry, start again from step 1

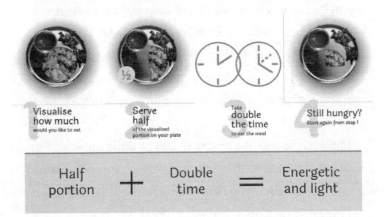

Visualise
how much
would you like to eat

Serve
half
of the visualized
portion on your plate

Take
double
the time
to eat the meal

Still hungry?
Start again from step 1

Half
portion
+
Double
time
=
Energetic
and light

Dates and coffee

Among the best things of my work are travel and a peek into cultures far and beyond. And the reassurance and reinforcement of the exact same common sense, nani–dadi wisdom across all ancient cultures.

On a visit to Jordan for a talk, I learnt that there is actually a rule to how many dates and Arabic coffee you can have at a time. So, of course, you must drink that one cup that your host offers when you arrive along with one date. But you should allow yourself the second only if you can have the third (date and coffee). Stopping at two or four or even numbers is not allowed.

This I felt was such a beautiful way of knowing where to stop eating and such a practical way of stopping before getting full. Even yoga says that you should leave about 25% of your stomach empty when you finish a meal but Jordan shows you exactly how to put that into practice.

FAQs

Q: Is the mental meal map only for main meals or can I follow it even when I am eating a fruit or drinking chai?

A: In an ideal scenario, you take this approach throughout. Stop eating before you are too full. You can start with the big meals and over a period of time you will find this practice comes in handy irrespective of what you are eating, like an auto-reflex. And we are the original cutting chai people, so culturally we appreciate the practice and are quite attuned to it.

Q: What if I like something, can I overeat?

A: Yes, by all means. Some chais or some samosas or some jalebis are so special that they deserve an extra bite. Eat it in a manner that allows you to celebrate the meal, long after it's over, like a happy memory. Here's what I always say to my clients, my secret rule to overeating really – did it lead to good conversation, sex or laughter or allow you to close an important business deal? If yes, then it was worth it. Celebrate it. And from the next meal, go back to living and eating normally. The key is to be aware of your appetite and to know when you have crossed the Lakshman Rekha.

Q: Why not just portion control?

A: Because appetite is a moving entity. Season, the state of your mind, where you are eating, who you are eating with, everything affects it. Even your workout intensity and quality of sleep will influence your hunger. So stay engaged with your meal and eat exactly as much as you need to, not more, not less. And over a period of time, even awareness becomes natural and effortless. Work towards it.

Alia and the two monks

After an unwinding trip in New York City, Alia was sitting in my office, telling me that she had indulged in too much food and a few drinks too. 'You had a good time, na,' I asked her. 'Time of my life,' she said. 'Toh, vasool then,' I said to her. She looked at me, confused. As a dietician, I should be playing the role of tch tch, bad girl, don't have a good time please.

'You heard the story of the two monks?' I asked. 'No,' she said. Two monks are on their way to the monastery and they are sworn to celibacy, goes the story. The monastery is in a jungle, on top of a hill, with wild streams to cross on the way. Near one such stream, the monks see a petite young lady struggling to cross the stream. One of the monks bends forward, carries her in his arms and drops her off at the other bank. The two monks then continue the journey, upwards and onward towards the monastery. As the hill approaches, the climb is steep, tough and an out of breath monk asks the one who carried the lady, 'With what face are you coming to the monastery? We are sworn to celibacy and you think nothing of carrying women in your arms.' 'But I dropped her at the bank and you are the one who's still carrying her,' replied the other.

'Shit, I should come here more often,' said Alia, 'and listen to your stories.' 'Come, putri, come. Food nahin, guilt is fattening.'

Week 9

Guideline

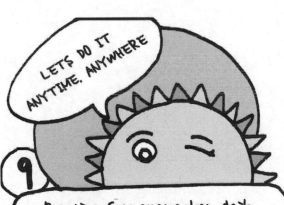

LETS DO IT
ANYTIME, ANYWHERE

9

Practice Suryanamaskar daily.
Choose a fixed place at home.
preferably a well ventilated one.
Fix a time to do it daily -
sunrise or sunset are good times.

The Guideline

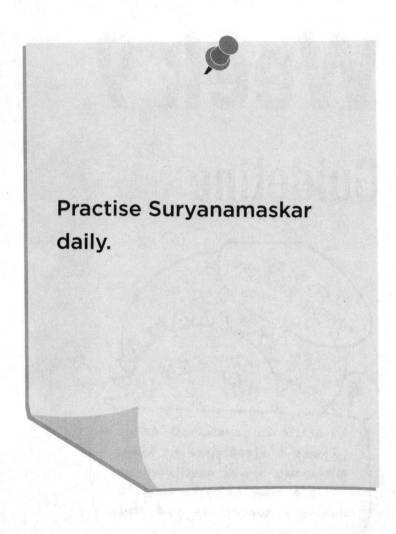

Practise Suryanamaskar daily.

Notes

We have only four more weeks together and by now you have already integrated eight lifestyle changes into your daily routine and here's the latest one. The one which has stood the test of time, the one that bridges the gap between strength and calm – the one and only Suryanamaskar.

In ancient India, it was a practice for children to perform five Suryanamaskars every day as part of the daily routine along with brushing, bathing, eating, etc. My grandfather or Ajoba died at the age of 87 around noon, but he had done his Suryanamaskar, dusted the house and eaten his lunch – routine was complete. He had a six-pack not because he wanted one but because it was inevitable.

Basics of Suryanamaskar practice

★ Choose a fixed place at home, preferably a well-ventilated one

★ Fix a time to do it daily – sunrise or sunset are good times or you can even fix your time as pre-breakfast or post-bath, whatever works best

★ Breathe normally and take your time to learn the correct posture, no rush

★ One on right, one on left together make one round

Video link:
www.youtube.com/watch?v=BOlydiuO50A

Benefits of daily Suryanamaskar practice

Fitness, broadly, has four components – strength, stamina, stretching and stability. You can call them the 4 S's of fitness. And the one form that engages with all the components simultaneously and without big investment of time, space or money is Suryanamaskar. You can literally do it any time, any place, and the only equipment you need is discipline. It's good for all ages, genders and all seasons. Regular practice of Suryanamaskar:

✓ Gives you a strong muscular back. Given our inactivity, poor posture, etc., we are losing the strength in the back which is required to keep not just the spine healthy but to connect the strength in the physical body, more specifically of the gluteus, to the strength or calm in the mind. If we feel weak in our body and aggressive in our mind it's because we don't have a strong back.

✓ Gives you ageless, radiant skin. This is not just a cosmetic benefit but a real reflection of good health. The skin is the largest organ of our body and if the skin is healthy it means that the kidney, liver, heart, all organs are healthy and well nourished.

✓ Hormonal balance. If there is one exercise that works directly on our glands – thyroid, adrenals, pituitary – it's the Suryanamaskar. From optimum metabolism, pain-free periods to healthy levels of vitamin D, the practice will ensure that the glands work at their best.

Special instructions to make progress

1. If you have never done Suryanamaskar before
- Start with 2 rounds every alternate day
- Graduate to 2 rounds every day from week 3
- Then add 1 round to your practice every alternate week

2. Do it but not very regularly
- Tie it to a non-negotiable; for example, won't leave from home without the practice
- 5 a day is a good number – sustain that
- If you feel like doing one more, wait for 12 weeks. Train the mind to be consistent first.

3. Doing it regularly
- Don't take a break even on a Sunday
- Don't drop below 5 or go beyond 12
- The idea is to get better with every step and not to mindlessly increase the number

FAQs

Q: What if it is too hot or I am feeling too tired?

A: On a day you are feeling too hot, too exhausted, too tired, just drop the right half of the round where the right leg leads. Just do your rounds on the left and see how light you feel.

Q: Should I do Suryanamaskar during periods?

A: Feel free to listen to your body. Do it if you are in good shape, drop the number if you are exhausted.

Q: How to modify in case of PMS issues?

A: Start with 3 full rounds and end with 2 rounds only on the left.

One full round of Suryanamaskar = Full sequence leading from right leg + full sequence leading from left leg

One round on left = Full sequence leading from left leg + repeat

Q: What if I have back/knee pain?

A: Focus first on the right technique. Skip the postures which aggravate the pain, but do the rest in sequence.

Week 10

Guideline

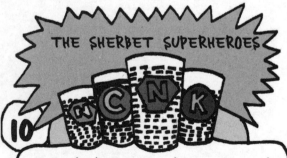

THE SHERBET SUPERHEROES

Have sherbets and other traditional summer drinks through the day. Some options - NARIYAL PANI - mid morning. BUTTERMILK - just after lunch. NIMBU SHERBET - with early eve snack. KULITH - for dinner.

The Guideline

Stay hydrated with sherbets
and other seasonal drinks
through the day.

Notes

Over the last few guidelines, we have been trying to expand the conversation about health and fitness beyond numbers, labels and food groups and we will now take it one step further.

One of the things we would traditionally do is change what we eat and drink as per the season. For example, you will notice that you either get lethargic, sick or fully acidic during summers. And the fact that you don't sweat as much in winters can make you inattentive to your thirst signals and leave you dehydrated.

But the good news is that it doesn't have to be like this. There are easy ways to ensure we stay at optimum health during different seasons, and this is the guideline for this week.

Some of the most popular traditional drinks and why and when you should have them:

★ **Nariyal pani – mid-morning. Preferably before noon**

Helps keep the acidity and acne down. And if you get enlarged pores in summers, then once or twice a week, add half a tsp of sabja seeds to your nariyal pani.

★ **Chaas (buttermilk) – just after lunch**

Other than being a good source of vitamin B12, this coolant will ensure that you are not bloated in the second half of the day. Especially useful if you take BP or diabetes medicines or are just recovering from a course of antibiotics. Also helps with sweet cravings.

★ **Nimbu sherbet – with your early evening snack**

Add salt, sugar, jeera and black pepper to your nimbu pani. There are many alternative sherbets also for summers – kesudo, wala, kokum, variyali, bel, etc. The body's natural AC, these micronutrient-rich sherbets won't let your electrolytes or water soluble vitamins drop, especially important if you are a BP patient.

★ **Kulith (horsegram) – at dinner**

If you have lost your appetite or feel low on energy or are simply feeling too gassy, this is what you need. Either make a dal out of it and eat it with rice, or turn it into a pithla (like a soup) with dahi and just have that for dinner instead (every region has a recipe for that). You will not just sleep better but also wake up with your skin feeling fresher and tummy flatter. Thanks to the folic acid and mineral-rich kulith, the super pulse of India. Also a very good option for those with diabetes or weak digestion.

★ **Amla sherbet and kaali gajar ki kanji**

These two drinks of North India are nutrient-packed and allow for a smooth transition from summer to winter. They ensure that you are not congested or coming down with a flu, just because the season has changed. These vitamin C- and A-rich drinks, along with their healthy bacteria, will even prevent the free radical damage that the body goes through when the pollution levels shoot up.

More about kulith

Eaten from north to south and east to west, this is one of the therapeutic pulses of India, especially for kidney stones. It's an inexpensive source of protein and you can make it into a soup and have it with a dash of ghee, or like a dal and have it with rice or cook it and mash it like a potato and turn it into a paratha.

Like all pulses, for best results, soak it, sprout it and then cook it. Especially good for pigmentation and skin dryness during menopause.

Benefits of these traditional drinks

The traditional drink of every season is invariably from the forgotten, underutilized species of the region. The Ayurvedic wisdom behind including these drinks during the day as a mid-meal or as an accompaniment to a main meal was to stoke the appetite, ease digestion and boost the immune system. They introduce diversity to the diet, allow you to celebrate the season and eat roots, flowers, leaves, etc., in a fun, colourful manner. Sometimes tangy, sometimes sweet, sometimes sour, these sherbets are a priceless treasure of every Indian kitchen. Some more benefits:

☑ Help reduce acidity and get rid of bloating

☑ Promote growth of healthy bacteria and nurture intestinal mucosa

☑ Give a smooth, flawless complexion

☑ Prevent UTI and fevers

☑ Relieve chronic body aches and pains

FAQs

Q: Apart from nimbu pani, nariyal pani and sherbets, what other summer drinks can we have?

A: Each region has its own, here are just a few more:

Ambil – mixture of spices with ragi (or nachni) in buttermilk or curd

Panna – the kachcha kairi (raw mango) drink garnished with kesar or aam porar shorbot which is the burnt mango drink Bengalis have in summer

Neera – the virgin palm drink that can cure everything from insomnia to eczema.

Some more summer drinks – thandai, nannari, kokum, buransh (rhododendron), sea buckthorn, nettle soup, bel sherbet, wala or khus, rose.

Q: Can I have sugar cane juice in summer?

A: It is ideally a drink for winters but if you are drinking it in summer, crush a bit of ginger into it and always drink it before noon and drink it super fresh, the minute the sugar cane is crushed.

Q: Some more options for winter?

A: • Instead of chaas (buttermilk), have lassi, either mid-morning or late afternoon

• Make kulith dal and have it with bajra for dinner. Okay to have with rice too.

• You can also have amla sherbet (morning time) and chyawanprash with milk, either to begin or end your day.

• Peanuts and jaggery or cashews and jaggery as a mid-meal.

Q: Fresh coconut water is not available, what are the alternatives?

A: Kokum, nimbu, ambil, panna, bel, even buransh, all these are available even when fresh coconut water is not.

Q: You mentioned kulith, but isn't it a heating food?

A: All pulses are traditionally harvested in the winter but stored and eaten through the year. Belonging to an ancient culture means that there is already a system in place to use them based on the season. So in winter you can have kulith paratha like they do in the Himalayan regions and in summer you use the same kulith but cook it with dahi or chaas and turn it into a cooling drink, like kalan in Maharashtra. In both seasons, it helps prevent skin ageing, increases Hb levels and helps boost immunity.

Our grandmoms spent centuries fine-tuning these recipes; it's our turn now to honour them and keep our cool.

Afghanistan

Kabul. I could write an entire book on the two days I spent there recently for my talks at the Indian embassy and the United Nations, but my main takeaway was haft mewa. A drink made with the choicest of local dry fruits, with a generous helping of shehtoot (or mulberry). This drink is the toast of spring and signals the arrival of flowers, warmth and of people drinking it on the roadside. Also a sign of optimism that all will go back to normalcy and peace soon. Sarve bhavantu sukhinaha (not inspired by Lady Gaga).

Week 11

Guideline

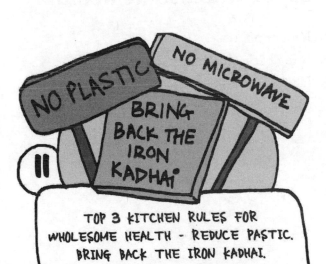

TOP 3 KITCHEN RULES FOR WHOLESOME HEALTH - REDUCE PASTIC. BRING BACK THE IRON KADHAI. HEAT. DONT MICROWAVE.

The Guideline

Follow these three kitchen rules for wholesome health

1. Reduce plastic
2. Bring back the iron kadhai
3. Heat, don't microwave

Notes

Any conversation about fitness actually begins from our kitchen. That's exactly the place from where health, harmony and happiness originate.

★ Reduce plastic. You can start with these easy steps:
1. Use cloth bags instead of plastic bags to shop for vegetables and fruits. Avoid buying veggies and fruits that come individually packed in plastic or thermocol.
2. No plastic tiffin boxes, especially for hot food, and no plastic cutlery, haath se khao. Also, no cling films for fruits and dabbas. France by the way is the first country to ban plastic cutlery. Use steel dabbas and malmal cloth for wrapping rotis, etc.
3. Use steel or copper water bottles when travelling and not plastic bottles (including mineral water bottles).

★ Bring back the iron kadhai – yes please, inse naata jodo.
1. Say bye to your Teflon-coated non-stick kadhais that have made you believe that

glory lies in avoiding fat (you know now that it doesn't).

2. Cook your poha, upma and sabzis in an iron kadhai. Don't forget to add ghee or oil and spices and I bet you will never fall short of iron ever again.

3. Also, let go of the aluminium vessels and foils too. You can use stainless steel, pital and other metals. Exposure to aluminium lowers the levels of zinc, an important mineral for our bodies, especially for brain health and preventing diabetes.

★ Heat, don't microwave. First of all, if you are microwaving, it means you are just overcooking and then overeating, followed by overstoring and again overeating. So stop this vicious cycle. If you have to heat food, simply heat it slowly on flame. Microwaving is harmful for the micronutrients in the food as it quickly heats them at extremely high temperatures where their bonds break and they get oxidized and become toxic for your body.

Socho mat zyada, go back to cleaning up your kitchen. And don't forget to involve the men of the household.

Why?

☑ Plastic is a major pollutant not just for our environment but also for the hormonal balance in our body. It releases estrogenic chemicals in our body and disturbs the ratio between our male and female hormones. Especially important if you have PCOD, adult acne or are a young girl at puberty.

☑ The iron kadhai is an important and undervalued source of iron in your diet.

A lot of lack of energy, enthusiasm and anger stems out of low Hb levels. Micronutrient deficiencies don't always need an expensive supplement, they just need an inexpensive change in the kitchen environment. Women who struggle with too much bleeding during periods or complete lack of it are often prescribed iron tablets. But then a lot of women are unable to take the supplement due to the digestion problems it causes. Simply changing to cooking in an iron kadhai solves this problem. Most of my clients who struggle with Hb levels and are barely able to maintain it at 9 see it climbing up to 12 once they switch to iron kadhais and tavas. You can make your bhakris, chillas, dosas on it or cook your dals and sabzis in it. Sometimes I wonder why in the world did we trade our lokhand, pital and tamba for aluminium, plastic, non-stick.

 Cooking – It is the unbroken thread of wisdom that links us to our past and takes us to our future. A lot of the progress we have made as *Homo sapiens* has got to do with the fact that we cooked food and made more nutrients available to our body and brain to fuel our dominance as a species. Cooking is underrated though, and this is where gender biases come into play. Kitchens are mostly the bastion of women, and the activities that happened in there are undervalued because of deep prejudices against women. But there is nothing lowly about cooking (or women). It takes a calm, collected and creative brain to cook a meal. And then one thing that New India should aspire for is boys who can cook – cook a hot meal for their spouses routinely and take pride in it. At every talk I give in schools and colleges, I tell girls that they must only date boys who can cook dal–chawal. If you ask me, a gender equal society starts from the kitchen. Pay attention to who, how and what is cooked in there.

FAQs

Q: I live abroad and mostly cook once a week and then eat it over the rest of the week. If not micro then what?

A: Bring out the portion you want to eat in a small vessel (buy some on your next trip to India) and then slow-heat it on your gas stove. It may take a minute or two more than microwaving but the nutrients and taste it retains is well worth the trouble. If you are unable to heat on a regular stove and microwaving is the only option, use a ceramic or glass bowl and avoid plastic. Every step in the right direction counts. And as you follow the guidelines, you will, over a period of time, find the energy to cook at least one more time in the week.

Q: When I make green sabzis in an iron kadhai, they come out looking black. Quite an eyesore – any ideas what to do?

A: Make the sabzi and then immediately transfer it into a glass or ceramic or mud bowl. The dark colour is just the addition of iron. It isn't a bad thing but putting it into another vessel right after cooking can help you keep its aesthetics too.

Q: What about khatta stuff like imli or nimbu or kokum in an iron kadhai? My dadi says don't use an iron kadhai in that case.

A: She's right. In case you are adding anything sour to the curry or dal you are cooking or even if you are making kadhi (that uses buttermilk, etc.), you can use a pital ka vessel with kalai (tinning) or even a steel ka bartan with a copper bottom. Consider using an iron karchhi, that's your grandma's method of adding iron when a kadhai was not possible. You have to dip the laddle once the dish is ready, leave it for a while and then remove it.

Q: No plastic but then what about boxes and bottles or high grade plastic for storing of lentils and grains?

A: You now get tiffin boxes and water bottles not just in steel but also in earthen ware, kansa and the like. Same with storage. You can also use glass containers for storing lentils, etc. The idea is to avoid plastic as much as possible. Even with fruits, when you cut them open, try to finish them by sharing them with all at home. Buy smaller quantities of fruits and vegetables to begin with and don't plastic wrap them. Just keep them in a small katori and cover it with a lid if you want to refrigerate the half-cut fruit.

Week 12

Guideline

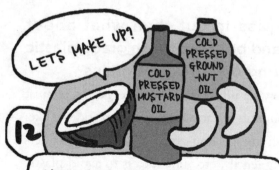

BRING BACK THESE 3 FATS IN YOUR DAILY DIET - TADKA IN KACCHI GHAANI OILS (COLD PRESSED). COCONUT AS GARNISHING, CHUTNEY, ETC. CASHEW AS A MID-MEAL OR WITH MILK BEFORE SLEEPING

The Guideline

Bring back these three fats in your daily diet

1. Tadka in kacchi ghaani (cold pressed or filtered) oils
2. Coconut as garnishing, chutney, etc.
3. Cashews as mid-meal or with milk before sleeping

Notes

So, well, officially, the last guideline but pyaar apna hamesha ke liye rahega just like aap ke khane mein swaad hamesha rahega. And it's fat which adds taste to your food, along with satiety, satisfaction and sustainability in the diet.

★ **Tadka in kacchi ghaani oils**
Use oils native to your region – mustard for North and North-East India, groundnut or til for central and western and coconut for Kerala. Our native recipes are fine-tuned to the fatty acid and nutrient composition of our oils and to make the best out of what we eat, we have to follow them in totality. No jumping on the bandwagon of 'heart healthy' or other such promises made by refined vegetable oils (rice bran, safflower, sunflower, soya, canola, etc.). Avoid oil free or fat free at all costs. And kacchi ghaani because then it means that the oil is extracted at a lower temperature and therefore fatty acids, vitamins and other nutrients are intact. Very important for diabetics to have traditional oils.

★ **Coconut as garnishing, chutney, etc.**
From supporting gut health to helping you calm your nerves to soothing digestion, there isn't a thing coconut can't do. The fact that it is antibacterial, antiviral, is an added bonus. If you are the type that gets UTI every summer, don't forget the coconut. So garnish your food with it, turn it into laddoos and barfis, make chutneys out of it, have the coconut malai and even the dry coconut with jaggery or just peanuts.

★ **Cashews as mid-meal or with milk before sleeping**
Other than the good fat, cashews are rich in minerals, amino acids and vitamins. The amino acids help, among other things, in the production of serotonin, the natural sleeping pill whose only side effect is a stable, happy mood the next day. The magnesium helps the nerves to relax. Its tryptophan (an amino acid) and vitamin B combination help make kaju a natural antidepressant. It's the summer nut and you can eat the cashew fruit too (super rich in vitamin C). (More details in my book *Indian Superfoods*.)

The reason I stress on cashews is that they remain underutilized due to the misinformation around them. They are as healthy as almonds or walnuts, if not much more, but they don't have an industry association supporting them.

Why?

Essential fat is required for both the body and the functioning of the brain. Without adequate fat in our diet:

☑ We won't be able to assimilate vitamins like vitamin D, minerals and other essential nutrients from our diet

☑ We won't produce the right hormones and may suffer from weak joints and nerves. This role that fat plays is especially critical for children.

☑ Blood sugar will stay unregulated and there will be cravings for sweets after a meal

☑ Skin can age prematurely due to lack of nourishment from food

FAQs

Q: How is cooking in traditional oils and ghee beneficial for diabetics?

A: Cooking in traditional oils is a marker that you are eating more traditional and time-tested meals. It is well known that the main challenge with diabetes is unregulated blood sugar. Meals that are adequate in ghee and oils, the ones that are not shy of calories or essential fatty acids, are low in the glycaemic index and have a beneficial effect on blood sugar. They also help in fat loss and prevent skin pigmentation.

Q: Belong to North India but staying in South or vice versa. Which oil to use?

A: Depends on what you are cooking. If you are cooking a regional recipe, use the regional oil and if you are making a traditional dish, use the one you grew up eating.

Q: I live outside India, what are my choices?

A: First of all, your health food stores are now full of ghee or clarified butter and, really, Indians abroad are in a way spoilt for choice. So you can pick up cold pressed groundnut oil, sesame oil (when winters are harsh), coconut oil, mustard oil – based on what region of India you originally belong to.

Q: Is cashew okay for high BP patients?

A: Yes, it is. It's rich in minerals that help dilate the blood vessels, making circulation easier and BP more stable. And yes, it has zero cholesterol.

Edible oil

All packaged and processed foods have this ingredient. Invariably it comes from palm oil. The palm oil industry has led to major deforestation in biodiverse forests but because the prices are low and because of the versatility of the oil, it continues to thrive. You will find it in almost everything – pizzas, lipsticks, chocolates, shampoos, etc. It has put endangered species like the orangutan and Sumatran rhino at further risk. Recently an awareness campaign 'there's an orangutan in my bedroom and I don't know what to do' was banned by Iceland. It aimed to create awareness about how palm oil production was shrinking habitat for animals already at risk of extinction. The thing is that the more we move away from our native produce for cheaper or even 'healthier' alternatives, the more we eat into what is not ours. And at the end of the day our health is entwined with that of the rhinos, bees, elephants, snakes, etc. The approach that we take towards health must be a sustainable one not just for us but for all those that Pashupatinath of Kathmandu looks after, that is, every living being on earth. Long story short, eat within your environmental means and look beyond the food industry narrative of carb, protein and fat.

And that's it folks,
12 weeks over,
12 guidelines done.

Chapter 4

How to get to forever: The 12 steps

Remember that the diet rage of today is going to be the garbage of tomorrow and the best way to be on a diet is to never get on one. It's like how they say that the best way to stay in love is to never marry;) Or at least to not put yourself in the role of a husband or a wife. Because roles are often limiting, not just for you but even for your partner, reducing you to what you are not, assigning you a specific task and then leading to a stage we are all familiar with, that search for 'myself' or 'I need to do something for myself', the quintessential mid-life crisis.

Food should be viewed for what it is, a blessing. And a blessing should be accepted in all its glory, not in divisions and ratios of carb, protein and fat. The wrong attitude can reduce the biggest blessing to a curse. Food or anna can lead to a path of self-discovery, unfolding the mysteries of life, and liberate you from all attachments and fear. One where, if nothing else, you are free from forcing your body to fit itself into a certain size. One where you are free to enlarge your life and not decrease your size. When you truly begin to understand what food is in all its glory, the journey to forever, beyond this body and lifetime, begins.

But gyan apart, if I had to summarize the fitness project into 12 learnings or steps that allow you to make the journey from now to forever, this is what I would say:

- Food is nourishment, security and opportunity to grow
- Grow and patronize local food
- Local food is climate-resilient
- Resilience is much more important than weight loss
- Loss of energy and enthusiasm is a big price to pay for being skinny
- Skinny is not a sure-shot way to success

- Success comes at every size
- Size doesn't matter to people who matter the most
- Most of the people spend a lifetime chasing things that they never even wanted in the first place
- Place strength, stamina, stretching and stability at the core of your workout routine, not calories
- Calories are dead, declared the *Economist*
- Economists, ecologists and agriculturalists (and of course farmers, tribals, dadis and nanis) know more about food and well-being than most dietitians, doctors and trainers.

And finally the cliché, but a relevant goodbye line – a journey of a thousand miles starts with just one step. So even if you have missed out on a few weeks, start with that one step, as many times as you have to. And always acknowledge how far you have come. And don't worry about the journey ahead, it's going to be a good one. Keep your head down and walk. Walk the path of joy, health and fitness. One step at a time.

Appendix 1: Some references for the 12-week fitness project

Arredondo, A.; Azar, A.; and Recamán, A.L. 'Diabetes, a global public health challenge with a high epidemiological and economic burden on health systems in Latin America'. *Global Public Health* 2018, 13: 780–87.

Büssing, A., et al. 'Effects of yoga on mental and physical health: A short summary of reviews'. *Evidence-Based Complementary and Alternative Medicine* 2012: 165410.

Food Planet Health, Healthy Diets from Sustainable Food Systems. Available at https://eatforum.org/content/uploads/2019/01/EAT-Lancet_Commission_Summary_Report.pdf

Jung, S.I., et al. 'The effect of smartphone usage time on posture and respiratory function'. *Journal of Physical Therapy Science* 2016, 28: 186–89.

Lee, H.Y., et al. 'Metabolic health is more closely

associated with decrease in lung function than obesity'. *PLoS ONE* 2019, 14: e0209575.

Nicklas, T.A.; O'Neil, C.E.; and Fulgoni, V.L. 'Rice consumption is associated with better nutrient intake and diet quality in adults: National Health and Nutrition Examination Survey (NHANES) 2005–2010'. *Food and Nutrition Sciences* 2014, 5: 525–32.

Nicklas, T.A.; O'Neil, C.E.; and Fulgoni, V.L. 'Snacking patterns, diet quality, and cardiovascular risk factors in adults'. *BMC Public Health* 2014, 14: 388.

Njike, V.Y., et al. 'Snack food, satiety, and weight'. *Advances in Nutrition* 2016, 7: 866–78.

Park, J., et al. 'Waist circumference as a marker of obesity is more predictive of coronary artery calcification than body mass index in apparently healthy Korean adults: The Kangbuk Samsung Health Study'. *Endocrinology and Metabolism* 2016, 31: 559–66.

Pem, D.; and Jeewon, R. 'Fruit and vegetable

intake: Benefits and progress of nutrition education interventions: Narrative review article'. *Iranian Journal of Public Health* 2015, 44: 1309–21.

Sharma, H.; Zhang, X.; and Dwivedi, C. 'The effect of ghee (clarified butter) on serum lipid levels and microsomal lipid peroxidation'. *Ayu* 2010, 31: 134–40.

Stefan, N., et al. 'Identification and characterization of metabolically benign obesity in humans'. *Archives of Internal Medicine* 2008, 168: 1609–16.

Stefan, N., et al. 'Metabolically healthy obesity: Epidemiology, mechanisms, and clinical implications'. *Lancet Diabetes & Endocrinology* 2013, 1: 152–62.

Thompson, R.C., et al. 'Plastics, the environment and human health: Current consensus and future trends'. *Philosophical Transactions of the Royal Society B: Biological Sciences* 2009, 364: 2153–66.

Westcott, W.L. 'Resistance training is medicine: Effects of strength training on health'. *Current Sports Medicine Reports* 2012, 11: 209–16.

Appendix 2: Feedback from participants

Rekha B. S. – End of first week, energy level increased, PMS irritations reduced, definitely.

Aparna B. Asthana – Hi, I am a typical example you had quoted – one with sweet cravings post each meal and very low in energy post lunch/ evening hours of the day. In fact recently had thought of going through medical check-up as well. However, started the banana first thing every morning and I have seen a drastic change. With NO sweet cravings at all and same energy level throughout the day.

Mubeen Amina Azam – I have not craved for anything sweet for lunch, even with sweets at my reach, haven't had them, it's a big achievement, what a simple banana can do.

Tanisha Tanisha – I have stopped craving for tea now which I just could not live without.

Loveena Bajaj Salve – Following week 2 guideline I absolutely love it. No hunger pangs in between meals and no sugar cravings throughout the day.

Jyoti Bhate Chhabra – I am loving the ghee part, it's yum and I am already feeling energized and the feeling of fatigue is gone.

Dr Farheen Khan – I am a medical doctor myself and used to fear ghee like ghost! I started with it and feeling so much better now.

Bhawna Arora – My all vital organs are thanking you for re-reminding us of ghee. It's been two days only while following this tip and already my stomach is calm and feel full. And lesser time in washroom with feeling of getting fresh first thing in morning, it's such divine feeling.

V. Sneha – I started following both tips from week 2 and I have stopped craving for sweets after meals. Thank you very much for knowing exactly what our bodies need and making us pay attention to ourselves with small changes in day-to-day life.

Preethi Swami – I had my first gadget-free meal in ages! I never understood when people said food should be a sensory joy. Today, I got it. Without any distraction, my breakfast looked good, smelled great and tasted fabulous!!!

Smita Oberoi – Maintaining the posture is the most difficult part but worth all the effort. Trying my best to follow it sincerely!! Meal without gadgets is a wonderful experience when all our senses are alert and active.

Richa Ranjan – Reading this on PC. My mobile use has gone down by 50% since your week 3 guideline. After 8 p.m. mobile is only to receive important calls, no other business.

Neeta Kanani – I'm following all the guidelines, they are amazing. Didn't know when they became a habit. Gadget-free before bedtime habit superb, I spend time with self. Results are reduced stress and dreams are clear, deep sleep and positivity.

Chitra Chandrasekaran – Guideline 3 works well for dinner time. It really helps in portion control.

Pragati Pandey – I started following your 12-week guidelines at the start of this year. My period and PMS issues were terrible at that time. Now at the end of the year, I am realizing how simple my life became after following the guidelines. My PMS issues are gone and I got 11 periods this year, which is a huge achievement for me. I have never felt better.

Dr Vaishali Chikhalikar – I am experiencing a great change in myself since I followed the fitness project. My TSH was 9.14 in Dec. Now today I rechecked after successfully completing the 12 guidelines and it is 7.97.

Subhasri Srinivasan – I have tried to follow all your guidelines and I am continuing them as much as possible. I noticed reduced bloating from the first week itself. I had been diagnosed with adenomyosis in Oct '17. I suffered from a lot of menstrual pain during my periods, to the extent that I had to take leave and stay in bed for at least one day of the period. It also caused indigestion and constipation for the second half of my menstrual cycle. After the everyday intake of badam/raisins with saffron, I noticed that the bloating and indigestion have reduced to a huge extent.

And in my last period, the pain had significantly reduced! I thought I would have to suffer with the pain throughout my life. But with my last period, I have hopes that if I keep following your guidelines, make informed choices with my food and lifestyle, I can overcome this issue.

Shanthala Nagesh – I used to face heavy bleeding during my periods from past 8 years. Thank you so much, from the last 2 months it's just very normal.

Varsha Gugale – I am following all the guidelines. I started eating rice dil khol ke. You won't believe but I have lost 5 kg since the last 2–3 months. I have started feeling energetic throughout the day. No period pain, initially my legs were paining after sunset, but now no more pain, only health gain.

Priya – I would like to mention that the sweet cravings that I used to get have vanished after I started having a spoonful of ghee and jaggery after lunch and dinner.

Sunita Zende – Thank you so much for initiating fitness project 2018. I have started sleeping like a baby, thank you so much.

Dinnah Moraes – I love to read, even while eating.

So, following that guideline about being gadget-free during mealtimes was AN ACCOMPLISHMENT! I slipped up a few times, but I now eat quietly. And what a DIFFERENCE it has made! I automatically eat less and savour my food more. I am involved with the family conversation while eating (not lost with my head angled towards my phone, mindlessly shovelling food in my mouth). And of course, I now don't use any gadgets an hour before bedtime and it's helped me sleep better and, more miraculously, wake up automatically without an alarm! Wonders never cease.

Izza Gul – For me reducing gadget time and not looking at it half an hour before I sleep has made a lot of difference. I always felt half asleep in morning but on second day when I started avoiding gadget before sleep time made huge difference, and I was shocked to know this minor thing was having major effect on my general daily activities.

Devleena Das – We, both husband and wife, are following your fitness project 2018. Usually I suffer from acid reflux but many thanks to you it's now under control due to the banana and 4–6 p.m. wholesome food.

Suchitra Gokhale Javalgekar – Eating banana/ raisin in the morning, snacks during 4 to 6 p.m. and ghee in three main meals – no sweet cravings, increasing energy level so regularity in exercise, reducing sleeping problem.

Anomita Bhaumik – Huge improvement here. I've always enjoyed walking but never enjoyed taking the stairs because I used to get out of breath after a few steps. Apart from the health aspect, I've also often suffered from this mental laziness, where I'd take a taxi to many destinations (vs public transport) by justifying that I'd get late. But after reading the guideline, I was able to make a mental shift where I decided to take public transport everywhere possible and this meant that I was 'planning ahead' and not making excuses. Due to the inclusion of public transport in the majority of my daily journeys, I started taking all the stairs (or walking up the escalators vs standing still) that came in my path. All of a sudden, I can do 15–20 flights of stairs every day without any hassle and in fact have even done 40+ flights of stairs on certain days. Now standing still on the escalator feels lazy and odd to me.

Nisha M. – It's been nearly 4 months since I started following your guidelines. Thanks to you for making me understand the mistake that I was doing. And also, I have learnt to listen to myself. I give exactly what my body needs (fresh and local food regularly, 30 minutes of exercise per day regularly, right sleep). Today I have no complaints of catching cold or throat infections.

Meghana Raikar – This is awesome and it feels so good to do strength training. The more weights I lift the more confidence I get and want to do a bit more each time.

Shreyasi Sharma – I can't thank you enough for opening this opportunity that everyone could be healthy and happy. Being a patient of PCO, I now understand the importance of strength training.

Jyoti Luthra – I was not doing my weight training but I started after the guideline. I have gained 2 kg of weight after weight training but:
1. I am very energetic.
2. I don't feel suffocating while doing workout.
3. I have lost inches from my tummy, as it's not now projecting as a bulge.

4. When I stand straight my tummy is looking flat.
5. And I can now sit crossed leg, which I didn't used to be.

Anjali Nair – I used to be 78 kg when I started and around 40 inches around waist. I started noticing visible changes in 2 months' time. Then I moved with my husband and all my dreams of becoming fit went for a toss coz managing a toddler without help is a big task and there is no time for anything else. Still, I held on to the dream and followed what all guidelines I could. If I were to estimate in this whole year my percentage of following the guidelines was just 40% roughly, still the results are just amazing.

Nikhila Lanka – I am a California resident. And I recently came to India for vacation. I followed your 12-week guidelines and I have become thinner and I am fitting in my two-year-old clothes. I don't measure my waist in inches or use a weighing scale. I just followed the guidelines blindly. And I found out that I was thinner only after coming back home. Never knew becoming thin is such an effortless task.

Neha Bhatia – To be very honest, when I started following your fitness project 2018 guidelines, I did with an open mind, but given how many attempts in the past I made, I did have my share of skepticism at the back of my mind. Nevertheless, I 'listened' to every word you said and tried to imbibe it. The result is that I have dropped sizes and now from wearing L down to M and the best part is all this has been CONSISTENT. I feel confident that it's not coming back. I feel confident going to tailor to get my dresses downsized and don't run the risk of not fitting in them again. (Incidental benefit is I feel I have a new wardrobe without spending a new penny :)) I don't run the risk of gaining all the weight back just because I got back from a short vacation (which I just did by the way and ate out all meals for 9 days but not gained crazy weight).

Rasshmi Mmahajan – I always eat white rice every lunch and dinner. Ghee is always there. Helped me so much with digestion and good news is zero bloating.

Purnima Mandal Shahi – Thanks for this! I have been having dal rice with ghee since few months now and it has improved my digestion and now I don't feel bloated.

Parul Lakhani – I am very happy to share with you that within 11 weeks of following your advice my blood pressure which was going out of control since last 2–3 years even with the tablet is now in control and I have stopped the tablet completely. Your super simple to follow instructions and advice is showing tremendous difference in the way I look and my energy levels have gone up considerably. I feel and look more young.

Shivi Goyal – Within 4 months of following your tips in the fitness project I had lost 10 kg of weight and since then my weight had been constant for almost 8 months.

Karuna Sahay – I can't even show my happiness to you. Finally, I am pregnant. I have conceived naturally. I have followed your 2018 guidelines and it works. Rujuta, I can't even explain how much this is important to me.

Priya Balijepalli – I haven't lost much of my weight (as yet). But the amazing things that are happening to me are:

1. Energy levels all-time high.
2. I can do 12 rounds of Suryanamaskars without going breathless . . . beat that!! Unlike the earlier times, when I would give up in 3 rounds. Nothing made me more happy than this!
3. I can play with my kid without complaining of tiredness.

Vibha Talati – Have been doing Suryanamaskar since this guideline first came out. Started with 4 and moved to 5. Loving the feeling and happy with the progress. And the best part is, it has become like a daily habit.

Sheetal Bhambwani – The 12-week fitness project was my first commitment ever towards any fitness programme. What transpired in the weeks to follow was my learning curve of my understanding about food, health and fitness. The simplicity of instructions to the point which can be incorporated into our life effortlessly for the rest of the life were the key winners to my mind. Surprisingly they yielded results pretty soon, for all the abuse that our body has been put over the last so many years. That kept me glued to follow the programme all through.

Neha Jain – I start my day with soaked and peeled almonds and soaked raisins. I have given up on aluminum and non-stick cookware as much as possible and adopted steel and iron ones instead. I do not store anything, even warm, in plastics. I have started eating ghee without guilt, I have added more dals and pulses to my diet and try to eat at least one serving of a dal/pulse every day, etc. I did not feel I had to do anything extra for adopting these tips but the benefit I have got from them is something I could never imagine.

Janhavi Dattawadkar Deshpande – I've started using iron kadhai for cooking and the food tastes awesome!!!

Akshata Rao – Following all your weekly routines I've lost more than 2 inches and 8 kg . . . that's really awesome.

Aishwarya Marathe – Since you've started the fitness programme 2018 I'm the happiest person. I used to feel so bloated before but now I feel so light and comfortable!

Nibedita Chatterjee – I love cooking and through my efforts I try and incorporate 12-week guidelines in my daily routine. In 1 year's time I have overcome my age-old gastritis and also my autoimmune disorder, which made me suffer for 7 long years.

Vaishali Chauhan – I followed all the suggestions and I did notice changes in me, not in just how much I weigh but how I feel now. Though on the scale I have noticed a change of 40 kg in 1 year and 7 months but I feel good about myself now (from 98 kg to 58 kg).

Appendix 3: The 12-week fitness project for kids and families

The 12-week fitness project for kids and families was conducted from January to March 2019. More than 20,000 families from across the globe participated and saw huge improvement in health and attitude towards food, especially in the children. The structure of the project stays the same – 1 guideline to be followed cumulatively every week.

Week 1 guideline: Healthy options to start the day for your kids

When our children wake up from an overnight fasting state what we feed them first will decide not just how good their entire day goes but also how their growth is. This meal is especially critical for children around puberty as it sets the tone for hormonal harmony.

In fact, how well they are able to unwind at night and fall asleep is also dependent on how they start their day. A nutritious, fuss-free meal then is of utmost importance.

Here are some options:

A. If short on time and can only have a quick meal before leaving for school:

1. Milk – if they like the taste of milk
Ensure that it is:
- Full-fat
- Locally sourced
- Without malted or chocolate powders
- With jaggery/chyawanprash (winters) or sugar/gulkand (summers) or a homemade laddoo
- No milk substitutes like almond milk or soya milk, etc.

2. Nuts and dry fruit
- Eat as nut + dry fruit combo
- Nuts – pista, almond, cashew, walnut
- Dry fruits – raisin, dates, khareek (dried dates), apricot
- If constipated – raisins soaked overnight
- Girls on period – khareek with ghee

3. Fresh fruit
   - Local
   - Seasonal
   - Banana all months
   - Bor, chickoo, peru, orange, grapes – whatever is currently in season
   - No fruit that has travelled more than 150 kilometres to reach your plate or comes in plastic packaging

B. If there is time to have a proper breakfast:
   - Have a hot, homemade nashta – poha, upma, idli, dosa, paratha, dalia, etc.
   - Nothing from a packet – cornflakes, oats, juices, etc.
   - If poor immunity – ragi cooked in milk or even water
   - If weak digestion, acidity or period issues – lahya, jowar or ragi flakes (look like popcorn) in milk or roasted in ghee with salt and pepper.

Also note:
   - Fathers must contribute to cooking, serving and watching over kids while they are eating

- Kids above seven years – pick own bowl/plate, rinse and put in kitchen sink

Remember, well begun is half the battle won.

Week 2 guideline: Peanuts and jaggery mixture right after school instead of biscuits/chips/chocolates

Our children often come back home from school feeling a bit low on energy. They are hungry and need something nutritious to eat. But this is also the time when they refuse to sit down and have a proper meal. This snack is the perfect solution for such situations, and ensures that they stay off junk food.

- It's handy
- Can be had in car, bus or while walking back from school or as soon as they reach home
- Allows kids to choose proportion of peanuts and jaggery as per their taste

Why peanut and jaggery?

- Complete meal, wholesome but not cumbersome to eat or even prepare

- A super mix of micro-minerals, vitamins and polyphenols
- Rich in essential fats too, good for the heart and bones. Especially good for athletic kids and gymnasts in particular.
- Extremely high in antioxidants, making it a boon for kids who don't like eating fruits
- Has the minerals and vitamin B profile that eases puberty and cramps during periods

Options
- You can use cashews instead of peanuts
- Add 1–2 tsp of ghee if your kid is allergic or low on immunity
- You can even garnish this with fresh coconut or eat it with a piece of dry coconut. Especially recommended for kids who are fighting obesity, diabetes or fatty liver.
- In summer, you can use ghee-roasted kurmura or lahya and mix peanuts with it instead of jaggery

Teach your kids to eat in sync with the crop cycle. This is the way to stay healthy and fit in the future too.

Week 3 guideline: Kids should play at least 60 minutes every day, even at the cost of tuition class or homework

Our children are not getting the basic minimum physical activity that is recommended for good health and that is one reason for rising rates of obesity, allergies and frequent illnesses in our kids. The World Health Organization recommends a minimum of 60 minutes of free play every day till the age of 17 years. Do note that more than 60 minutes brings additional benefits.

Regular physical activity:
- Leads to healthy musculoskeletal tissue (bones, muscles and joints)
- Leads to healthy cardiovascular system (heart and lungs)
- Promotes neuromuscular awareness (coordination and movement control)
- Facilitates maintenance of healthy body weight
- Improves psychological well-being, self-confidence, social interaction and integration

In the long term it also ensures that kids are less tempted to get into drugs, alcohol and smoking once they begin to experience the benefits of staying physically fit.

As parents/society we can facilitate physical activity for children by:

- Encouraging them to play in all weathers and seasons
- Teaching boys to share open spaces with girls and teaching girls to fearlessly occupy open green spaces to run, jump and roll in
- Allowing them to bunk tuition class or homework if it comes in the way of 60 minutes of free play
- Letting politicians know that free access to open spaces will get them your vote

Week 4 guideline: Fixed bedtime and wake-up time for good sleep

Do you find that your kid is getting sick often or is moody or cranky? Well, all she needs to do is develop good sleep hygiene. Essentially, habits that lead to good sleep. And the most important of those habits is to have a fixed time to go to sleep and wake up on most days of the week, if not all.

What's the right time to go to bed?

- Between 8 p.m. and 9.30 p.m. is ideal as this allows for optimum sleep
- Teenagers may extend it to 10.30 p.m. but not later
- Practise waking up at the same time every morning
- If your child sleeps much longer on weekends, know that they are sleep deprived
- Remember that you can't make up one night's sleep by sleeping too much the next day
- Overall, sleepovers are not a cool idea. Restrict it to once or twice a year.

Why is sleep important?

- It helps protect from all NCDs – obesity, diabetes, fatty liver, etc.
- Improves academic performance and creativity
- Reduces stress and anxiety in teenagers
- Supports growth and strengthens immune response
- Improves memory and deletes all that is unnecessary
- Improves EQ and all mental health issues like ADHD

Week 5 guideline: Wholesome dinner

Wholesome, simple dinner at least six days a week – dal–rice, khichdi, roti–sabzi. Forget variety for dinner.

What will you eat for dinner is a question that we should never ask our children. Instead we should tell them what they will be eating for dinner – a steady, simple and nutritious meal.

Three tests your dinner should pass:
1. It should be a meal that was your grandmom's dinner too
2. It should be local to your region
3. It should be easy to cook, and tastes best when served hot

All traditional combos like roti–sabzi, dal–chawal, khichdi–kadhi meet this requirement and it ensures that the growing bodies and brains of our children meet their requirement of nutrients too. It even ensures sound sleep. The key is to stay consistent with dinner, even at the cost of it being boring, on most nights of the week. And yes, don't forget to add ghee.

What you must not have for dinner on a regular basis:

- Variety* – different meals every day
- Ready-to-cook meals like noodles and pasta
- Takeaway or ordered in food

*You may offer your children variety for dinner once a week at home, ideally on a Saturday.

These do not have the nutrients to fuel growth, often leave our kids dehydrated and disturb the sleep routine too.

Eating out – Not more than twice a month, and that includes the times they may have eaten out because of birthday parties, etc.

Eat simpler, grow faster.

Week 6 guideline: No plastic dabba or aluminium foil for school lunch

Instead use steel dabba and malmal cloth. For water, use a steel or copper bottle.

Why?

- When food comes in contact with the material we pack it in, it picks up the qualities of that material. Especially true when we pack hot food.
- Plastic leeches a harmful set of chemicals called 'xenoestrogens' that mimic 'estrogen' hormone in the body and messes up the hormonal balance in the growth stage of our kids.
- Similarly, aluminium foils leech aluminium into the food and once inside the body, it replaces zinc, an essential mineral for insulin functioning. Impaired functioning of insulin leads to obesity and related NCDs like fatty liver, diabetes, PCOD, etc.

Essentially, we are packing our nutrient-rich food in cheap boxes and endangering the health of our children.

So while switching to a non-plastic source seems to be a small step, its health impacts are huge. It leads to:

- Reduction in constipation and illnesses
- Reduction in cranky behaviour
- Better skin, hair and nails
- Optimum growth and hormonal balance

Not to mention the huge benefit to our environment that reduction in plastic usage will bring about and we can hopefully leave a better world for our next generation.

Week 7 guideline: Healthy, tasty and easy lunch ideas

It seems simple but often becomes a daunting task to actually figure out what to pack for lunch. Kids easily get bored of eating the same food and sometimes we are just plain short on time to cook fresh meals. So here are some quick ideas that are healthy, tasty and easy:

1. Roti, jaggery and ghee – excellent for both the long and the short breaks. You can give a roti with jaggery and ghee on the side or have the child spread it and make a roll of it and you have a nutrient-dense dabba ready. Can even use last night's roti. Especially good in winters or when the kid is down with a cough, congestion or has low immunity. If your kid has frequent allergies, pick the liquid jaggery in winter. In summer you have the choice of roti with ghee and sugar or it's totally okay to continue with jaggery too.

2. Dahi rice/rice with tadka/fodnicha bhat/ vagahrelu bhat/lemon rice – easy to cook and tastes great even when cold. Rice typically doesn't taste great when it's not piping hot but thanks to its versatile nature, give it a vaghar or tadka or mix dahi and it turns into a great snack. You can pack the tadka rice with dahi or chaas that has hing or curry leaves along with a pinch of rock salt and you have a complete meal, which is also a perfect mix of pre- and probiotics. No yogurt in the market can match that. Good in all seasons, makes for a great big break snack or an after-school snack.

3. Fresh fruit – banana is my favourite, especially for growing kids, athletic kids and girls who get cramps during periods or if your kid's knees hurt in the evening. Rich in minerals, packed with vitamin B, this one is not to be missed on. Also, don't turn a blind eye to the ber, guava and amla that are in season or the mango, jamun, seetaphal, karvand when they come. Diversify your kid's fruit portfolio and put them on your teenager's plate. Don't buy into the marketing of kiwis, berries and the like. From constipation to acne and everything in between, the local, native fruits are a perfect cure.

Week 8 guideline: Practise asana, especially Suryanamaskar, daily

Children should practise yoga asanas, especially the sequence of Suryanamaskar, every single day. Usually the asanas and their flow in Suryanamaskar are modified to keep it more dynamic. However, advanced practices like pranayama, kriyas, etc., should not be done by children.

There are plenty of benefits of daily asana/ Suryanamaskar practice for kids. They:
- Lead to stronger bones and joints
- Inculcate a sense of discipline
- Calm the mind and get rid of restless energy

Note: Especially important for teenagers and children nearing puberty as Suryanamaskar is the one exercise that works directly on our glands – thyroid, adrenals, pituitary. From optimum metabolism, pain-free periods to healthy levels of vitamin D, the practice will ensure that the glands work at their best.

Children can start the practice of asanas and Suryanamaskar from age seven. Five

Suryanamaskars every day is a good number, and don't do more than 12. Can be done in the morning or evening around sunset.

Note: *Yoga for Children* by Swati and Rajiv Chanchani, Iyengar yoga teachers, is an excellent reference book for asana and Suryanamaskar practice for children.

Week 9 guideline: Regulate screen time to fuel growth and prevent obesity

In three important ways:
1. No screens during meals – will ensure that the child learns to pay attention to food and stays in tune with the stomach. This will improve leptin sensitivity and prevent overeating episodes in the future. Will also instil the importance of mealtimes.
2. No screens at least 60 minutes before sleeping – will ensure a restful sleep which is critical for recovery and growth at this age. Hormones like the growth hormone can then do their job during sleep. Also, no TV in the bedroom as

there is a strong connection between having a TV in the bedroom and childhood obesity.

3. Less than 30 minutes of total screen time daily – this can exclude homework assignments on the computer. Studies show a strong link between screen time and craving for junk food, especially sweetened beverages like colas, packaged juices, etc. Also, more the screen time, lesser the physical activity which can then lead to insulin resistance.

Week 10 guideline: Identify junk food and plan its consumption

Step 1 – Identify junk food
- Obvious junk food, which we can clearly identify as unhealthy, for example, fast food chains selling pizzas and burgers, packaged chips, colas, chocolates, ice cream, pastries, doughnuts, instant noodles, ketchup, mayonnaise, etc.
- Camouflaged junk food which pretends to be healthy but isn't, for example, breakfast cereals, juices (tetrapack, powders, etc.), biscuits (even the fibre-rich ones), dark

chocolate, chocolate syrups, malted powders for milk, cupcakes and muffins, ready-to-cook food, frozen food, energy drinks, baked or multigrain chips, jams and spreads, instant noodles (wheat, multigrain, vegetables, oats), flavoured yogurt and milks, etc.

Step 2 – Make a strategy for consumption

- Set a monthly limit. Ideally once a month. But if you are consuming a lot of junk food, plan to reduce by 50% each consecutive month. For example, if you eat junk food eight times a month, then in month one, reduce it to four, in month two, reduce it to two and in month three, reduce it to one.
- As parents, never give junk food as a reward or as a means of celebration (especially festivals) or to show your love. This leaves a long-lasting impact on impressionable minds.
- Always remember that your favourite superstars or cricketers who endorse these junk foods never have it themselves and only do it for money.

Why you must not eat junk food:

- It hampers growth – both physical and mental and ensures you never achieve your full potential
- It provides entry to all kinds of NCDs in your life – diabetes, obesity, fatty liver, PCOD, cancer and the like
- It leads to irritability, mood swings, loss of concentration, along with other mental health issues
- And worse, it is addictive. The more junk food you eat, the more junk food you will feel like eating. It's a vicious cycle.

Week 11 guideline: Learn and practise balancing regularly

Balance is the ability to carry out daily tasks while maintaining a controlled body position. Balance and coordination activities should be an integral part of every child's life to ensure that they develop gross motor skills, and improve posture and even confidence.

There are plenty of easy ways to do that – skipping

rope, cycling, swimming, skating, dancing, martial arts, hanging on bars, yoga postures like hand stands, back bends, inversions, etc.

Know that balance comes easy at a young age but gets difficult as one gets older. So the earlier your child starts with it, the better. Dedicate at least a couple of hours a week to practising balancing activities. It will give them an immense sense of power, freedom and intelligence, both to the body and to the brain.

Benefits of balance and coordination activities:
- Improves concentration and alertness
- Improves muscle strength and joint mobility and flexibility
- Teaches kids how to take a fall and reduces risk of fractures in the long term
- Improves confidence and social interactions with peers

By the way, the sit and rising test (SRT) is now even used as a predictor of metabolic health and longevity.

Week 12 guideline: Identify and refer to food in your mother tongue

It helps establish a connection with culture and cuisine, differentiate local foods from exotic ones and reduce the harm from junk food advertisements.

Many of you complain that your child eats only junk food, demands colas, ice creams and wants pizzas and pastas over home-cooked meals. One reason for that is a disconnect between the language they speak (English) and their mother tongue.

We have now started calling foods as carb, protein and fat and not dal–chawal, achaar, poori, thayir sadam, etc. When we don't call foods by their local names we can never establish that connection with them. Allowing our children access to the rich heritage of food and well-being of our culture would mean first encouraging them to speak in their local language.

It's exactly for this reason that the UN has declared 2019 as the 'year of indigenous languages'. India reportedly has over 19,500 mother tongues and all of our traditional knowledge about health and well-being is hidden in those. The various dialects that we speak connect us to our culture and cuisine and teach us to eat in a climate-proof manner.

Benefits of speaking about food in mother tongue:
- It helps kids identify which food is local to their region and therefore healthier. Local food is ecologically smart because it has not travelled a long distance to land on your plate and is also good for your farmer or local economy.
- It also allows them to see through a lot of exotic foods that have no health, economical or ecological value, for example, quinoa, cranberries, kiwi, kale, soya beans, broccoli, rucola, etc.
- It prevents them from falling prey to junk food advertisements. When food is spoken about in a local language it beats the constant marketing that kids hear about food in English.

So let's start from the dining table. As a family, only use your mother tongue or local language to talk about the food you are eating.

Additional tips

Special tips for summer vacations:
- Increase daily playtime to at least three hours
- Get kids to participate in making pickle, papad, sherbet, etc.
- If travelling, can have pasta/pizza, etc., for lunch
- Can eat chatpata snacks between 4 and 6 p.m.
- Drink gulkand milk before sleeping

Special tip for birthday parties:

Serve only three food items – a freshly fried one + a wholesome one + a sweet – for example, samosa + poha + jalebi *or* bhajiya + poori aloo bhaji + shrikhand

Note on the Author

India's leading sports science & nutrition expert and public health advocate, Rujuta Diwekar is a vocal champion of using common sense and uncomplicating the act of eating right.

Her books have sold more than a million copies and continue to define the discourse on food and exercise in the country. She emphasizes a blend of traditional food wisdom and modern nutrition science for a healthy body and mind, best reflected through the mantra – Eat local, think global.

She is among the world's most followed nutritionists with more than 2 million followers and 100 million+ video views on social media.